THE MODERN BOOK OF YOGA

EXERCISING MIND, BODY AND SPIRIT

CONTENTS

BACKWARD BENDS
120

TWISTS AND STRETCHES
140

BALANCING ACTS
156

COOLDOWNS
174

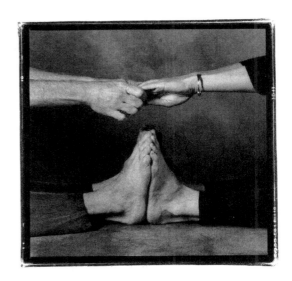

III
YOGA FOR TWO

AWARENESS SQUARED
185

DOUBLE HATHA
187

KUNDALINI PARTNERS
196

TANTRA
206

IV
INDEX
223

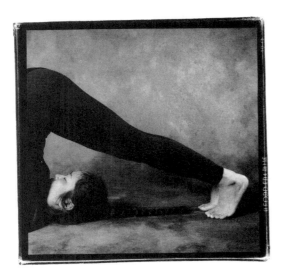

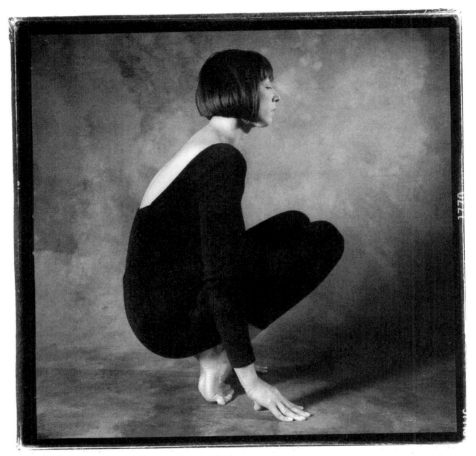

EXERCISING MIND, BODY AND SPIRIT:
STRENGTH IN UNITY
MEDITATION: REALITY TESTING
CHAKRAS, MANDALAS AND MANTRAS
BREATHING: AIR POWER

MIND, BODY AND SPIRIT

EXERCISING MIND, BODY AND SPIRIT: STRENGTH IN UNITY

If you want to change your body, change your awareness first.
—*Deepak Chopra, M.D.,* **Ageless Body, Timeless Mind**

Frost rimmed the windowpanes and wind rattled the tree limbs outside. But I felt warm and peaceful practicing breathing exercises on the living room floor of a chilly Boston brownstone at my first yoga class in 1968. Having pursued various forms of dance and exercise, I expected yoga to be another sport. The difference I experienced that evening changed the way I understood physical and mental development. I was inspired to study other Asian disciplines, from acupuncture to Zen, and later taught hatha and kundalini yoga in California.

Yoga is full of surprises. The first surprise was that it was not simply exercise. Yoga is a moving meditation, a system for developing the mind, the body and the spirit in unison. This holistic approach is what makes yoga feel different from Western sports training.

Another surprise is that those pretzel positions that look uncomfortable can feel like champagne. Yoga is not meant to be a spectator sport. Your attention is inward. Each pose is designed to awaken informative sensations in your body and to trigger a series of physical adjustments that improve your health. More surprises come over time as yoga offers an endless process for refining your physical and mental capabilities.

Yoga assumes people's mind, body and spirit need balanced attention in order to function fully. Modern scientific research on the interrelatedness of biological processes reflects this ancient wisdom. Richard Cytowic, a Washington, D.C., medical doctor, sums up current computer research on the human brain: "Some experts in artificial intelligence now believe that without emotion, thinking is impossible" (*The Man Who Tasted Shapes*, Warner).

Yoga combines three approaches to body/mind development: (1) exercise positions, or asanas, for toning the body; (2) breathing techniques, or pranayamas, for energy rejuvenation; (3) and mental development, or meditation, including mantra chants and mandala visualizations. Uniting these techniques for balancing mind, body and spirit is part of advanced yoga practice.

Ageless Benefits

Yoga can benefit people of varying ages and in various physical conditions. Children, too, have fun doing yoga. A beguiling book, *Yoga for Bears* (Richardson and Ward, HarperCollins SF) presents illustrations of a chubby cub in hatha poses. Perhaps your cub would like to practice along with you.

Athletic young adults are usually astonished at how challenging a workout yoga is because it appears relatively effortless. Most Western forms of exercise emphasize stressful movement of the muscles and the misguided "no pain, no gain" attitude. Yoga avoids harsh movements that trigger the production of large quantities of lactic acid in muscle fibers, which causes fatigue and tightness. Inhaling more oxygen lessens this fatigue, but it is not sufficient to counteract the negative effects of lactic acid. Rapid movement of the muscles also can cause excessive strain on the heart.

Thus, extreme muscle development is not necessarily a recipe for health. A healthy body requires balanced flexibility, stamina, strength, organ functioning and mental control. In yoga, movements are gradual, often slow, always paired with their kinetic opposites, and coordinated with complementary breathing and relaxation. After assuming each yoga pose, you hold the position alertly for as long as it is comfortable. This adds a crucial isometric aspect to yoga and builds muscle strength without pounding or tearing. You can become very strong without losing suppleness, injuring yourself, or suffering negative side effects.

One main reason to exercise is the health benefit of increased oxygen and blood circulation. Slow movements combined with deep breathing achieve improved health better than jerky, fast ones. Efficient, coordinated movement develops as one practices yoga, because the balanced poses improve the central nervous system.

Yoga is terrific for aging bodies. The most common early indication of physical aging is stiffening of the joints. Fluid movement is often thought to be the province of the young. But yoga can counteract this trend by careful attention to moving all the joints during exercise and keeping ligaments flexible. Faulty alignment of the spine and poor balance can cause shortening of the ligaments and many other movement problems. Yoga exercises keep your spine in good alignment, and the low impact of yoga movements prevents strain to muscles and bones. Yoga exercises also target glands and organs with movements that improve blood flow to those areas to ensure better cleansing of toxins.

Your degree of health and flexibility, not your age, determines how much you do. You should do only what feels good. Beginning yoga is practicing a comfortable version of the pose until your flexibility increases and your abilities and positions will become more advanced. Your measure of excellence is the skill and enjoyment at your own pace. As physician Deepak Chopra (*Ageless Body, Timeless Mind*, Harmony Books) points out, stress causes most of what we think of as signs of aging. Yoga lowers your biological age and reduces stress so your body can function well and look better at any age.

BIOLOGY IS FLEXIBILITY

Women may have an easier time than men as beginning students of yoga because they are less apt to have practiced years of heavy body building sports that shorten the tendons, flex primarily in a single direction, and leave one muscle-bound. Also women's hip joints are set farther apart than men's and can rotate in such a way that women often assume positions like Squat and Lotus with relative ease. This can be embarrassing to an otherwise athletic male student. Competition is not part of yoga. You measure your progress only by your own sense of fulfillment. Of course, an overdeveloped sense of competition can spoil a workout for a student of either sex.

Max Strom, an experienced athlete, has some encouraging words for brave beginning students who belong to a category he dubs, "the stiff white male." In an article in the magazine *Yoga Journal* (June 1995), Strom assures his fellow stiff males that yoga practice doesn't stay painful. "If you swallow your pride and work at a sensible beginner's pace, studying consistently, in a short time it will no longer feel like medieval torture. In fact, there are few things I've found to be more pleasant or rewarding. And eventually, eventually you will reach your toes."

If You Have a Guru Phobia

Some people are deterred from studying yoga by the mistaken idea that they need to believe in an Indian religion and wear saffron colored robes. True, diverse religions have adopted yoga as a tool for their own exploration and many gurus, or masters, such as Iyengar, have given their names to their schools. But basic yoga is not tied to any religion or to any guru. "Yoga philosophy does not quarrel with any religion or faith and can be practiced by anyone who is sincere and willing to search for the truth," states Swami Vishnudevananda (*The Complete Illustrated Book of Yoga*, Harmony Books).

There is a nondenominational, spiritual point of view at the center of yoga, which is a belief in a universal creator. Truth is defined as the realization that people and all creatures are part of the divine spirit. The aim of every yoga exercise is to give us a glimpse of this state of unity. Living as though we are part of a divine whole can free us from much suffering and confusion. But yoga does not ask you to accept this on blind faith. It offers down to earth techniques so you can feel a powerful wholeness in your body.

Unity of Opposites

There are many different yoga schools today. Kundalini practices deep breathing and strenuous exercises. Astanga, outlined in *Power Yoga* (Beryl Bender Birch, Fireside), combines variations of hatha postures with its own form of breathing and continuous, fast paced movement. Tantra focuses on couple exercises and sexual energy. Raja heightens spirituality by subduing body sensations in order to allow the mind to dominate. Although the philosophies may differ, the movements are largely the same. This book explores hatha yoga, founded on the idea that our bodies are not barriers but doorways to spiritual awakening.

In Sanskrit, hatha means "sun and moon," symbols of natural opposites. Yoga means "union," and is defined as the suspension of the mind's activities by means of breathing and balanced postures to unify our spiritual consciousness. Asana means "to sit with." These words together describe the yoga process of observing nature's opposites in order to understand unity.

Yoga can include highly intellectual study. The more you read yoga philosophy, the more it sounds like modern physics with the viewpoint that opposites form a natural unity. This connection is explored by Fritjov Capra in *The Tao of Physics* (Shambhala). Rodney Yee, a San Francisco based yoga teacher, describes yoga as "an alchemical process by which we develop awareness and self-control so that gradually we act more in accordance with our beliefs. We can live our philosophy, not just talk about it."

Yoga philosophy is an important part of training. But as you proceed, focus more on practicing the exercises than on thinking about the ideas. If you do, you will feel your changes, not just conceptualize them. The basic focus of yoga is to forge beyond words and meditation to understanding and action.

MEDITATION: REALITY TESTING

The body should be properly controlled by an intelligent driver, the mind. Prayer, and discrimination between the real and the unreal, will train the mind as an intelligent driver.
—*Swami Vishnudevananda,* **The Complete Illustrated Book of Yoga**

Knowledge is the true organ of sight, not the eyes.
—*Panchatantra, c. 5th Century*

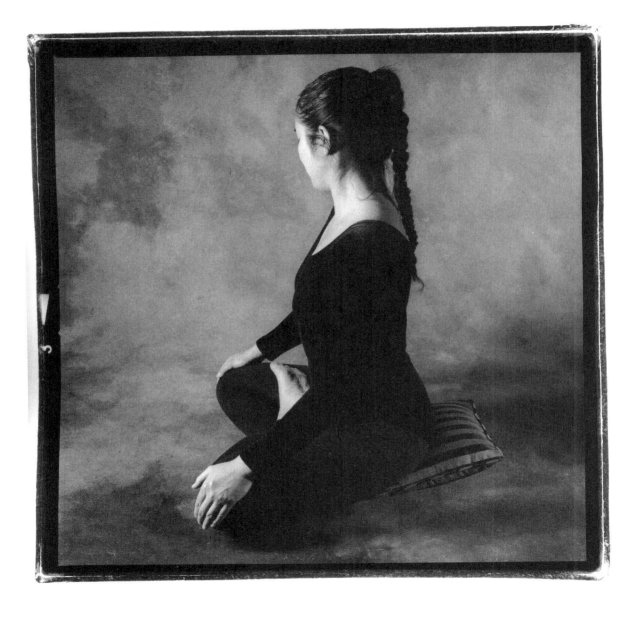

THE REAL THING

We are such stuff as dreams are made of.
—*William Shakespeare,* **The Tempest**

Meditations are like stretching exercises for the mind. When you start with them, everything that follows works better. The process helps you empty your mind of surface thoughts so that deeper, more profound perspectives can float into consciousness. Meditation allows us to relax and slow down our thoughts. The gaps between our thoughts become longer and longer. It is during the gaps which are free of judgment and emotion that we find peace and clarity.

In yoga our conscious thoughts are considered to be mostly confused, dreamlike misinterpretations or subjective distortions of reality. We become able to recognize spiritual truth, or reality, through the stages of meditation. And yogis believe that truth shall make you free.

The mind is a body part and needs exercise to function well. Use it or lose it.

SPACE EXPLORATION

Every solid particle of matter is composed of 99.999 percent empty space.
—*Deepak Chopra, M.D.,* **Ageless Body, Timeless Mind**

Meditation is the exploration of the pauses between thoughts. The mind can find balance that is considered more real, that is, more divine than thinking. This spiritual harmony beyond thought is described in the biblical phrase, "the peace that passeth understanding."

If you can observe your thoughts as neither good nor bad, just there, and identify with the calm between your thoughts, your moods and perspectives will become more balanced. Practice a meditation method, such as Counting Breaths (p. 24) for as long as you want. When you arrive at an alert, expansive peacefulness, remain in this space without using a meditation method. Resume the method only when you become distracted by thinking.

EMBODY YOUR UNDERSTANDING

The choicest fruit of meditation is that your participation in the world becomes more peaceful and constructive. See if you can develop the same nonjudgmental response to others that you are cultivating toward yourself during meditation.

EASY POSE

Honest.

A comfortable meditation pose for almost anyone.

1. Form a simplified version of the Lotus position on the floor by resting your feet, one behind the other, near your thighs.

2. Tuck a small pillow under the base of your spine to give your back a lift into straightness. Don't worry if your knees seem high. As your hip joints loosen, your knees will relax down.

3. Close your eyes. Relax your breathing, and focus on your favorite meditation from the following pages.

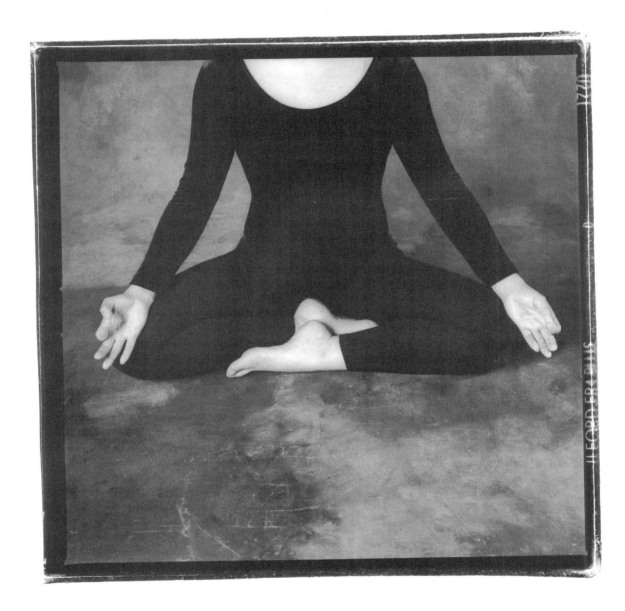

MEDITATION PILLOW

A proper lift.

1. Sit comfortably with your legs crossed loosely and your palms resting on your knees.

2. Place a firm, slim pillow or mat under your tailbone. This will afford your torso the slight lift forward that it needs to straighten, rather than curve backward.

3. When you have found the proper lift, you can sit without holding up with your muscles. The alignment of the vertebral column will support you without muscle effort and you can relax more deeply.

4. If you prefer kneeling and sitting on your heels, you can also place a pillow between your hips and calves for a similar lift. A small pad on the floor under your anklebones adds to the comfort.

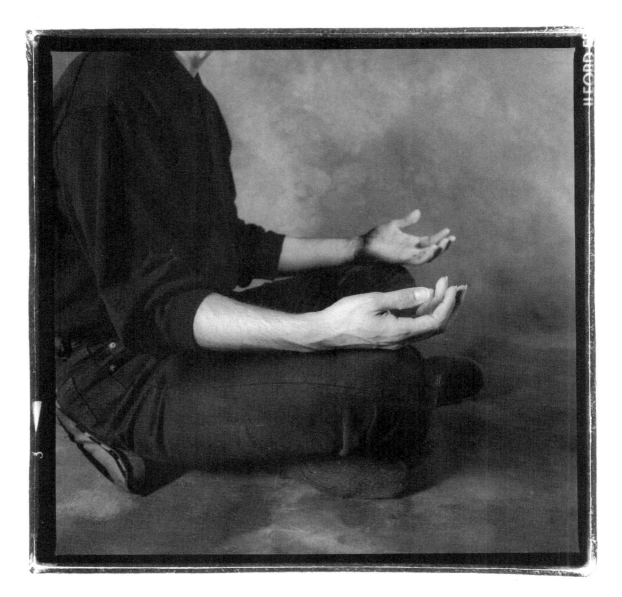

FULL LOTUS

▄▄▄▄▄

The mind blossoms.

In Indian mythology, the lotus flower represents magnificence coming out of mire. Because the roots are in the mud, but the head of the blossom always reaches for the sun, the white flower has become a symbol of spiritual enlightenment.

The classic Full Lotus position involves resting the tops of the feet on opposite thighs near the hip joints. This requires strong legs and advanced flexibility and should not be done until you have been practicing less taxing variations for a long time. Other versions, such as Easy Pose, Half Lotus, Double Lotus, and Relaxed Blossom, are also good for meditation. The Full Lotus is thought to be excellent for meditation, because it seals your body energy into a loop and intensifies your practice.

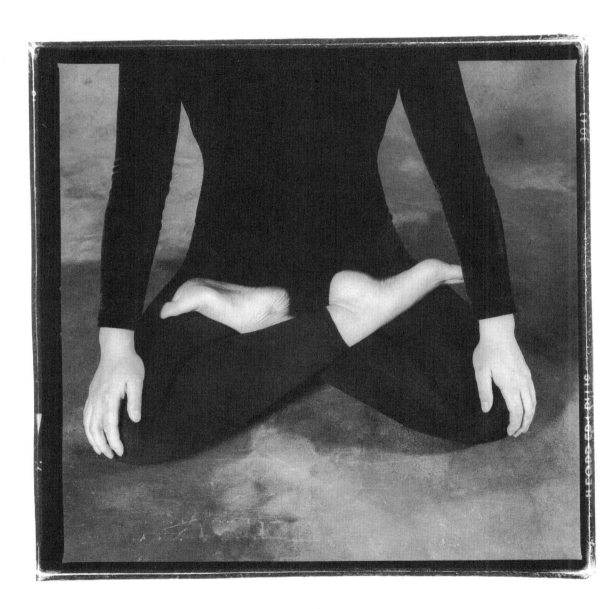

HALF LOTUS

■

A bud.

1. Sit on the floor with one leg extended; the other, with knee bent.

2. Place the foot of the bent leg up on the opposite thigh as close to the hip joint as is comfortable.

3. Fold the other leg under the upper thigh of the bent leg.

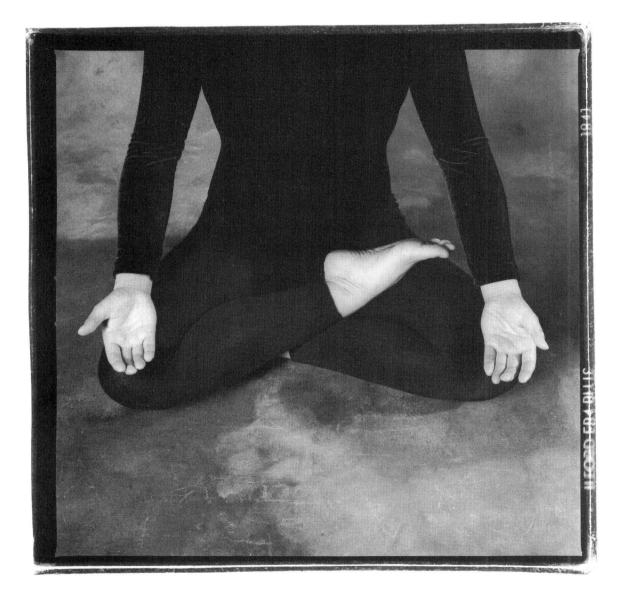

RELAXED BLOSSOM

Petals wide.

Sit with both knees bent and your feet tucked in front of your thighs so that the toes are pointing in opposite directions and the tops or sides of your feet are relaxed on the floor.

DOUBLE LOTUS

A garden.

Sit back to back with your partner. Meditate together and notice how another person affects your awareness.

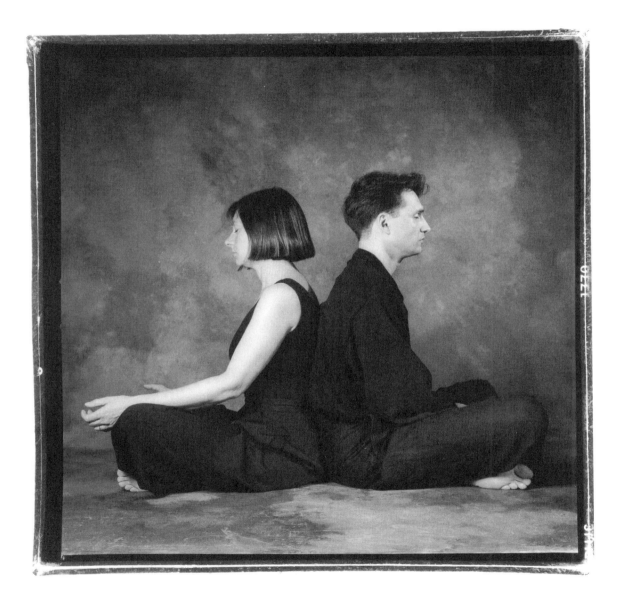

COUNTING BREATHS

████████

Awareness by numbers.

This simple meditation, which is taught to beginning students, can be one of the most powerful.

1. Sit spine erect in a comfortable position, such as Easy Pose or Relaxed Blossom. Close your eyes and place your hands palms up on your knees. Relax your breathing so you feel muscle movement low in your abdomen rather than high in your chest.

2. Begin counting your breaths. Consider an inhalation plus exhalation as one cycle; the next inhalation and exhalation is number two, and so on. Try to hold this focus without being sidetracked by other thoughts until you reach number ten.

3. If you got there without your mind wandering or losing count, you're probably an enlightened monk. At ten, start over

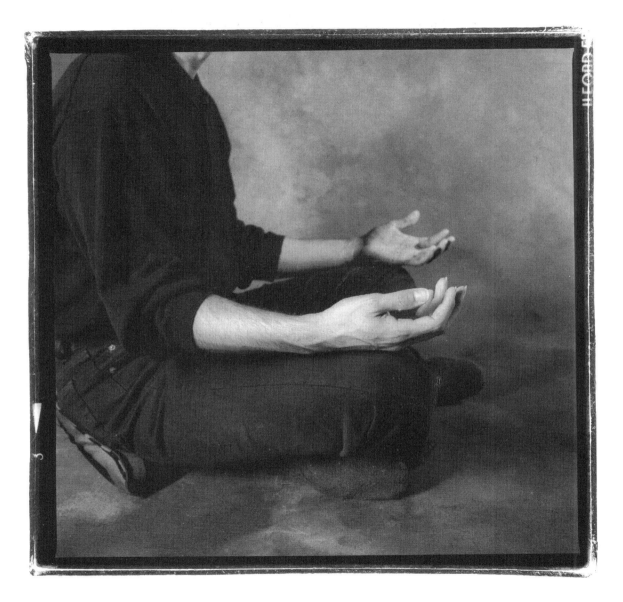

with one and count ten breaths again. Continue this cycle for a minimum of ten minutes. Work up to longer sessions.

4. A significant weeding out of mental static is going on as you count and concentrate. It can be helpful to imagine the thoughts moving across a film screen, passing into and out of view. Try not to linger with the thoughts. Just notice them, let them pass, and return to counting breaths. Gradually, the thoughts will be spaced farther apart, and the periods of neutral focus will grow longer. Don't judge the content. We all have a thousand ways to distract ourselves from our deeper purpose.

5. After a while you may notice that when you're relaxed you pause at the end of your exhalation. Enjoy this and allow it to lengthen. Thoughts will become less frequent as you focus your attention on the slow exhalation and gentle pause.

HAND MUDRAS

████████

Meditation Tips.

    A mudra is a position designed to unite the opposing vital energies in the body and keep them from separating. Bandhas, or locks, contain this energy inside the body. In yoga, the body is considered the vehicle given to us by the greater power for realizing spiritual consciousness, so care and respect for physical health is part of spiritual practice.

    The architecture of the body is seen as a conduit for various natural energy circuits. Each yoga posture is designed to focus electromagnetic and nerve currents to different parts of the body. These exercises can be used for specific health purposes as well as for mental awakening. Attention is paid to the positions of the hands and feet, as they are directional pointers, or turn signals, in the body's circuitry.

PALM SPHERE

A world in your hands.

We have modern technology that can locate and measure electromagnetic currents in the body. Centuries ago, yogis felt these subtle currents during their practice and included systems for directing them in their asanas to deepen the energizing effects of the movements. You can do a simple exercise with your hands to feel these currents. The experience offers you an additional aspect to your practice and helps you better appreciate how each detail of a yoga posture is calculated to heighten the power. Try this technique with your hands. Later you can try directing the energy to any part of your (or someone else's) body.

1. Sit comfortably, eyes closed, hands resting palms up on your knees. Relax any tense muscles you feel by imagining that each time you exhale, a little more tension leaves your body. Allow your breathing to be low in your body so your belly puffs out a bit as you inhale and sinks back in as you exhale.

2. Now imagine what it would feel like if you could send your exhalation through the center of your body, through your torso, to massage your muscles from the inside. Allow your breath to bring warmth and air to any tight areas. As you

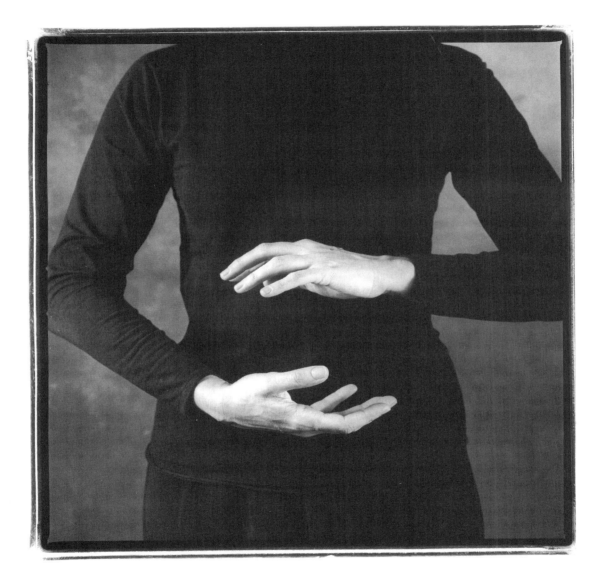

breathe, oxygen is drawn into your body and is spread to various parts through your bloodstream.

3. As you exhale imagine you can send air down through your shoulders and arms and eventually into your hands. What would it feel like if you could exhale down your arms and out the center of your palms through a spot about the size of a quarter?

4. Raise your palms so they are facing each other at about waist height. The increased circulation to your hands as a result of your breathing sometimes brings a sense of warmth and tingling. The muscle relaxation and improved circulation allow the body's electrical currents to move more easily. Can you feel any sense of this electrical flow between your facing palms?

5. Some positions intensify the current flow. Allow your hands to move slowly in any direction they want. Try holding them

different distances apart to see where the current feels stronger and where it weakens. You may sense a flexible shape to the air space. Sometimes it feels as though you are holding a ball between your hands.

6. The more you relax and direct your breathing down your arms, the stronger the sensation will become. You will notice that this process releases tension in your shoulders and arms. You can use this directed breathing to relax tight muscles in other parts of your body.

7. Healers learn to intensify this electromagnetic current so they can send relaxing sensations to other people. You can also experience the exchange of these natural currents during Yoga for Two exercises (starting on page 183). Being able to send and receive this energy gives you a resource for reviving tired muscles and spirits.

CHIN MUDRA

■■■■

Energy index.

A mudra position unites opposite body energies.

CHIN POSE Resting the back of your wrist on your knee as you sit in a meditation posture, press the tip of your index finger against the tip of your thumb. The circle formed is meant to keep the vital prana energy (see page 58) within your body by forming a loop.

CLASPED HANDS Another position to keep the vital energy circulating in your body is simply to relax your hands with the palms toward you in your lap with the fingers interlaced.

COVERED OR OPEN PALMS Resting your hands palms down on your knees as you meditate forms relaxed closure of the energy circuit.

Resting your hands on your knees with the palms open and facing upward creates a different circuit of energy, inviting input from around you and allowing your energy to flow back out again.

RIGHT AND LEFT Facing your partner, your right palm is positioned down and your left is up, resting on your knees. Your partner's palms mirror yours when you are doing a couple exercise. The right hand is thought to send out energy more readily than the left, which receives. In tantra couple postures, the palms of the partners usually meet according to this pattern.

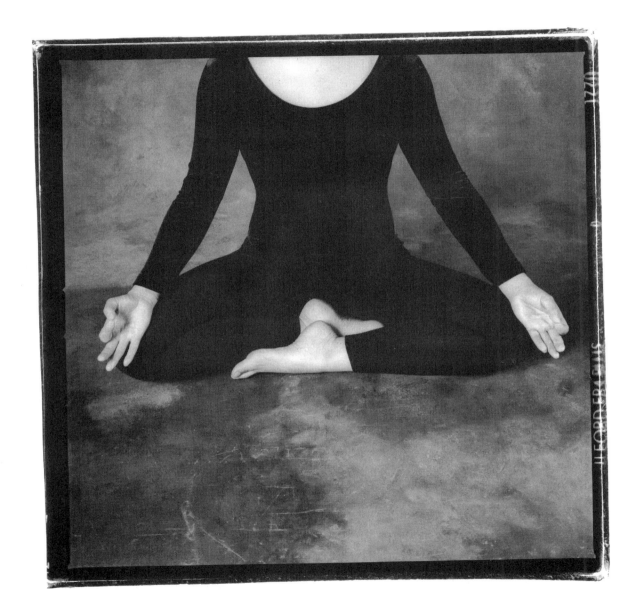

CHAKRAS, MANDALAS AND MANTRAS

CHAKRA MEDITATION

I think of the body as an electrical circuit that can become overloaded by the intensity of modern life. Yoga strengthens body and mind, enabling us to handle the intensity. Clarity comes when we allow experiences to flow through us rather than to build up tension and resistance.
— Rodney Yee, yoga teacher, San Francisco.

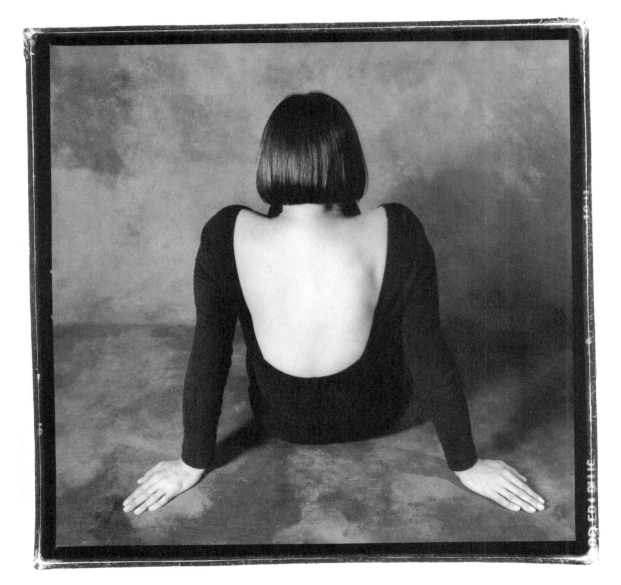

CHAKRAS: GRAND CENTRAL STATIONS

The word for a biological nerve plexus, or center, in yoga terminology is chakra. Each nerve center is thought to be a junction for spiritual as well as physical energy. A specific perception is attributed to each plexus that corresponds to a biological function. All centers need to be functioning well for the body and psyche to be in balance. A classic meditation is to start with the center at the base of the spine and relax each higher area and its associated function as your focus rises.

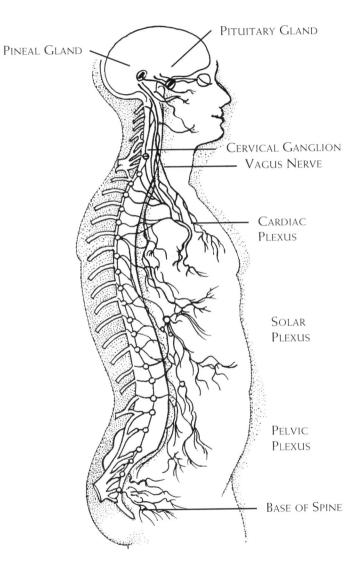

PINEAL GLAND

PITUITARY GLAND

CERVICAL GANGLION
VAGUS NERVE

CARDIAC
PLEXUS

SOLAR
PLEXUS

PELVIC
PLEXUS

BASE OF SPINE

CHAKRAS AND NERVE CENTERS

1. BASE OF SPINE: KUNDALINI CHAKRA. Starting point of the body's life energy and seat of basic molecular health and balance.

2. PELVIC PLEXUS: SEXUAL CHAKRA. Origin of erotic passion and biological creation.

3. BELLY PLEXUS: NAVEL CHAKRA. Center point of physical and spiritual balance; sense of self and inner calm.

4. SOLAR PLEXUS: ACTION CHAKRA. Diaphragm; channel for outer-directed power.

5. CARDIAC PLEXUS: HEART CHAKRA. Center of compassion; can infuse all other chakras with this aspect.

6. VAGUS NERVE AND CERVICAL GANGLION: THROAT CHAKRA. Communication.

7. PINEAL GLAND: MENTAL CHAKRA. Third Eye, or center of clear, rational perception.

8. PITUITARY GLAND: SPIRITUAL CHAKRA. Top of head; sense of perspective and unity; symbolized by the Thousand Petaled Lotus.

Traveling Light

In advanced meditation, the student combines breathing and chanting with meditation in an attempt to move the physical spinal, or kundalini, energy up from the base of the spine to the top of the head. Partial movement of this kundalini energy produces partial perception and stunted awareness. All the centers must be awakened and unified to produce full spiritual understanding and action. This is a gradual process that can take years, and the state of mental union can come and go. Someone who maintains this state of spiritual balance all the time is considered enlightened. Most of us see the light only briefly, but even small moments of clarity can illuminate a life.

Centering

Allow the fulfillment to come to you, gently resisting the temptation
to chase your dreams into the world.
*—Maharishi, **Unconditional Life***

Centering is a process of drawing the disparate influences around you into a unified order by focusing your attention on one thought or picture. From the resulting state of internal harmony, you can have a calm perspective to see events and emotions more clearly. Centering can be accomplished through various physical and mental exercises that bring opposing elements into perspective, so that they are perceived realistically as parts of a whole.

Mandala designs are visual aids for centering. Combining a seen mandala and a spoken mantra chant in your mental meditation involves multiple senses and thus intensifies the power of the centering experience.

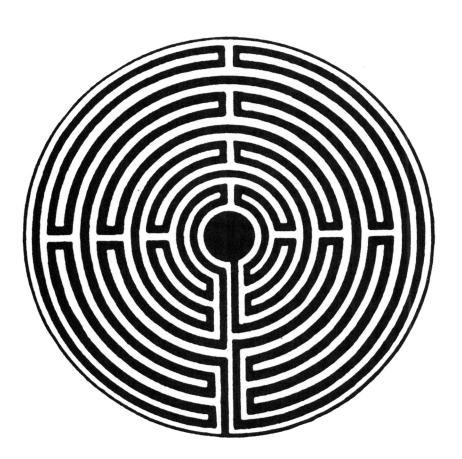

CENTERING

■

Coming full circle.

1. Sit in a comfortable meditation posture. Place a mandala picture, like the ones in this chapter, an inch or so below your eye level in the center of your vision, at least four feet away from you on a table or footstool. Jose and Miriam Arguelles explore painting your own picture in their book, *Mandala,* Shambhala.

2. Gaze steadily at the central area of the mandala image without allowing your eyes to blink very often. Allow your breathing to stay relaxed in your lower abdomen.

3. Maintain this gaze as long as is comfortable. Even though your eyes remain focused on the center, you will notice that visual changes occur in the areas of the picture in your peripheral vision. After a while, however, your vision will become more focused on the central spot. The center symbolizes the source of life energy. Try meditating on this concept as you gaze. Notice how your thoughts and vision change as you meditate.

MANDALA MEDITATION

If wholeness can be recognized by how it feels, the appropriate feeling is fulfillment.
—*Deepak Chopra, M.D.,* **Unconditional Life**

CENTER YOUR OPPOSITES

A mandala is a blueprint of the architecture of the natural world. In Sanskrit, mandala means "center" and "circle." Mandalas consist of circular geometric forms that suggest the concentric patterns making up all levels of life forms, from the cell to the solar system. From the snowflake to the cyclone, natural systems rotate around a central energy point. The center of the mandala design symbolizes the mysterious, inexhaustible source of all creation.

Mandalas are usually very beautiful, but they are not designed primarily to look pretty. They are designed to stimulate spiritual awakening in us as we concentrate on the center and allow our perceptions to align with the concentric patterns. The psychologist Carl Jung used mandalas as therapeutic devices for calming his patients. Painting them and gazing at them are meditation rituals.

Any balanced concentric form can function as a mandala. Several are shown here in simple line form. If color is added, more senses are awakened. You can study the symbolism of Asian colors or create your own symbolic cosmos. The male and female mandala symbolize opposite elements in all of us that bring unity when balanced within ourselves and in the outside world.

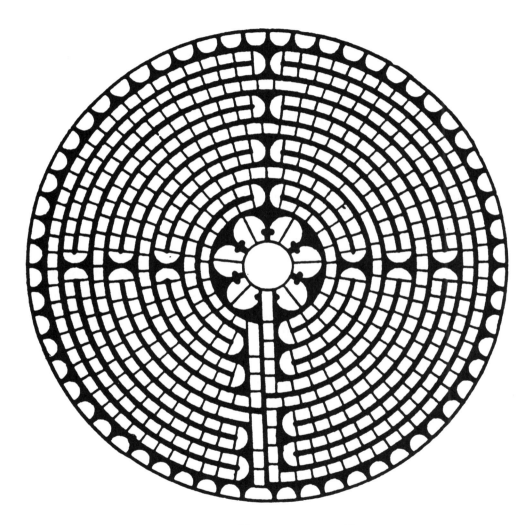

LABYRINTH IN CHARTRES CATHEDRAL

CLOCK FACE

■■■■

Take your time.

1. This exercise strengthens the eye muscles and improves the eyesight. Start with brief sessions and gradually increase the length.

Sit in a comfortable meditation pose with spine erect. Close your eyes.

2. Imagine your face has a clock painted on it. Keeping your lids closed, look up as far as you can at a spot in the center of your forehead where the number 12 would be on the clock. Hold this gaze for a count of five.

3. Shift your gaze a bit to the right as though you are looking at the number 1 of the clock, about the middle of your right eyebrow. Hold this gaze for five seconds.

4. Shift your gaze to the far corner of your right eye where the number 2 would be. Hold the gaze for about five seconds.

5. Continue around your face in a clockwise direction, stopping at each imaginary number until you reach 12 again.

6. Then reverse the process and gaze at each number in a counterclockwise sequence. Rest a moment with closed eyes, then open them slowly.

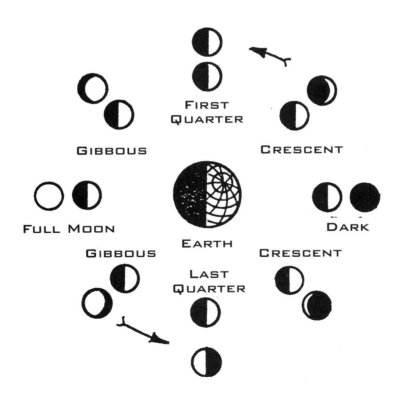

FLAME

Relax by candlelight.

1. Sit in a comfortable meditation position with spine erect. Place a lit candle about four feet away from you on the center of a table, so the flame is about at the level of your chin.

2. To develop concentration, strengthen the eyes, and clear the mind, gaze at the flame steadily for one minute without blinking.

3. Then close your eyes, relax your muscles, and for one minute visualize the flame inside your head between the eyebrows.

4. Repeat this sequence up to four times. As your eyes become accustomed to the steady gazing, you can increase each segment to three minutes.

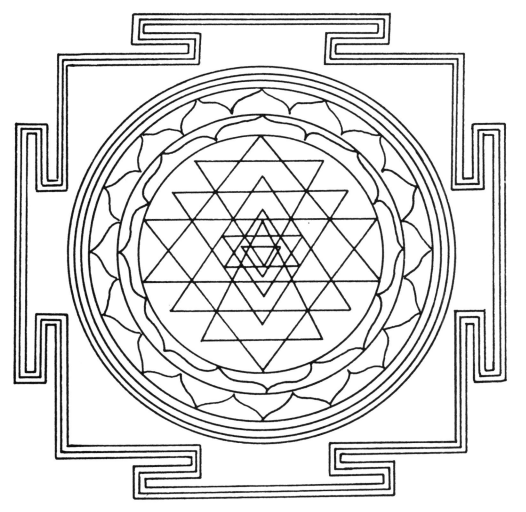

SRI YANTRA. FOR MORNING MEDITATION. MALE SYMBOL.

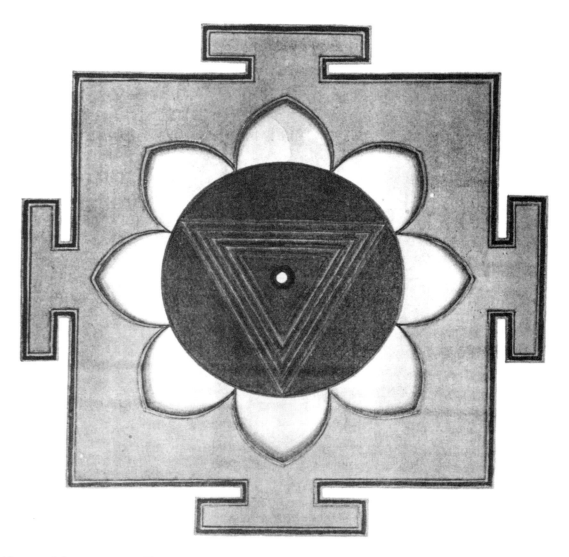

KALI YANTRA. FOR EVENING MEDITATION. FEMALE SYMBOL.

MANTRAS

SPIRITUAL SOUNDTRACKS

God respects me when I work, but He loves me when I sing.
—Rabindranath Tagore

A mantra is a mind song to soothe the savage body. The definition of mantra is "that which protects the mind." A mantra can be one of the names of God, or simply a symbolic syllable, which is repeated in thought, or a sound to stimulate spiritual awakening. Sounds with different pitches have frequencies that resonate in different parts of the body. Sounds can be combined to reach the areas of your choice. Play yourself like a harp.

SINGING WITH WHALES

Chants and mantras can sound silly to our ears if we are not trained to understand and hear them. We are usually expecting the melodic tunes for storytelling or dancing. Listening to or chanting mantras is like experiencing whale songs, which we feel in vibration more than hear in melody.

Knowledge
Whose substance is all mantras.
Reality
Whose nature is the true bliss.
Endless one.

—Vishvasara Tantra, **Tantra Art**

GIANT MANTRAS AND SMALL RAYS

Mantra syllables are traditionally Sanskrit alphabet letters, which symbolize different qualities, or Sanskrit words, which form a prayer. Sanskrit is the ancient sacred language of India. Mantras originated by certain teachers become identified with their authors. The mantra known as the Diamond Mantra is the mantra of the Buddha Padnasambhava. When we chant his mantra, we are saying his words, and it is thought that we invoke his powers of blessing as we do.

The two mantras of Tibetan masters that follow are long sentences or prayers. A single holy word can also form a complete mantra, such as the mantra "Aum." Not only does reciting mantras help heal ourselves, it also benefits others as the sounds spread in waves through the air.

THE DIAMOND MANTRA

OM AH HUM VAJRA GURU PADME SIDDHI HUM
(OHM AHH HOOM VAHJRAH GOOROO PAHDMAY SIDDY HOOM)

This mantra builds your power to act with strength and compassion in a difficult world, to function with diamond clarity.

> OM: clear body.
> AH: clear speech.
> HUM: clear mind.
> VAJRA: diamondsharp truth.
> GURU: wisdom.
> PADME: lotus symbolizing compassion.
> SIDDHI : realization or blessing.
> HUM: may this come to pass (similar to Amen).

Chanting this sequence of words repeatedly for as long as is comfortable invokes the healing blessings of the divine spirit. You are requesting God to give you clarity in all your aspects so you can act with compassionate power in the world.

THE MANTRA OF COMPASSION

OM MANI PADME HUM HRIH
(OHM MAHNIH PAHDMAY HOOM HREEH)

This mantra purifies negative emotion to transform it into our true, wise nature. Heals anxiety, negativity, confusion, and ill health.

OM: enlightened body.
MANI PADME: enlightened speech.
HUM: enlightened mind.
HRIH: active compassion (propels healing out to others).

AUM CHANT

All roads lead to Om.

The Vedanta Sutra sacred text from around the 5th century B.C. defines reality as that which persists in all circumstances. Most of the time we are caught up in changing ideas and pursuits. But now and then we see through surface illusions and have insight into more lasting perspectives. Yoga divides our average, muddled mindsets into three categories—waking, dreaming, and unconscious—all of which present distorted views of reality. Reality in yoga is the perspective beyond our personal viewpoint when we feel unity with the divine and see everything as part of this whole spirit.

The Aum Chant is an exercise designed to trigger this universal perspective through the repetition of sacred symbolic sounds of three Sanskrit letters. OM is the phonetic English spelling of the chant.

AUM is the Sanskrit word whose letters stand for:
A: the self in this material world,
U: the dream or psychic realm,
M: the unknown unconscious.

Chanting these letters together in the sound AUM can help unite our perceptions so that we experience a sense of our place in the larger cosmic order. The chant takes time to peel away the many layers of our illusions of separateness. Why not start today?

BREATHING: AIR POWER

*Most of the energy for the body we get from the air we breathe, and not,
as is commonly assumed, from food and water.*
—*Swami Vishnudevananda*, **The Complete Illustrated Book of Yoga**

In yoga the human mind is viewed as an unsteady element at the mercy of external influences. It requires calming and internal focus to function well. We all know it's not easy to control our minds. Breathing techniques are effective brain regulators because we can program our nervous systems by altering our breathing.

You may have noticed that when you are physically active, your breathing is fast paced and moves muscles high in your chest. When you are quiet and focused, your breathing automatically slows down and sinks deeper in your body. If we intentionally change our breathing, we can induce a variety of mental states at will.

SPIRIT LINKS

Breathing is one of the few automatic, unconscious body functions that also can be controlled consciously. This makes it an exceptional tool for mental development. Magdalene Proskauer, the San Francisco therapist who taught me the Palm Sphere exercise, says, "The breath is a bridge to the unconscious."

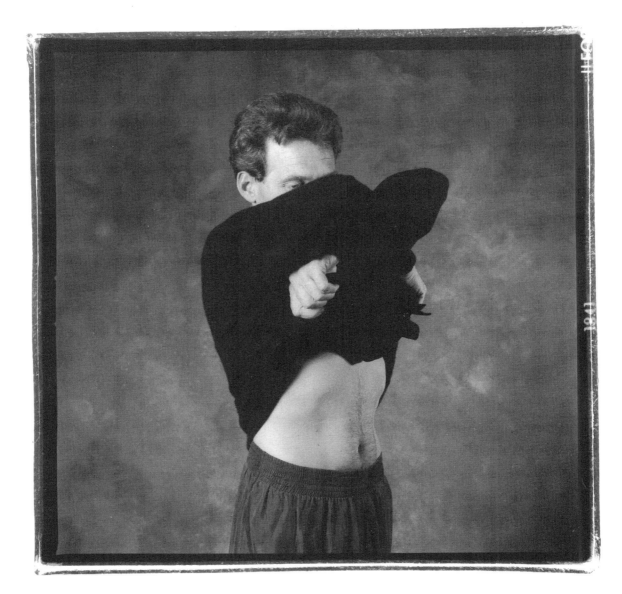

Every complete exercise system includes some breathing exercises. Yoga offers a spectrum of breath patterns for different purposes. In general, as you move through the postures, you inhale when you stretch and open up, and you exhale as you bend in and compress. The specific breathing patterns in this chapter are designed to improve awareness of the many parts of your breathing and to teach control over your cycles. The nostril breathing improves circulation and clears the mind. Some of the exercises tend to heat the body and some cool. Prana Seals, described later in this chapter, complete and intensify the effects of your exercise.

PRANA

Prana is the name for the energy current or life force in our bodies that animates all living things. Breathing is the result of prana movement. Our first and last breaths define our lifespans. When breathing stops altogether, it is evidence that the prana, or vital force of the body has departed.

Prana waves move in different patterns to produce every life form, from rocks and plants to people and ideas. Thought is considered the finest and highest manifestation of prana's movement in human beings. The process of controlling vital energy through breathing is called pranayama. The purpose of learning this control is to encourage the mind to higher planes of thought and understanding.

Prana is equated with life energy or vitality; thus, the more we have circulating in our bodies, the more healthy we are. The main storage area in the body for prana is the solar plexus nerve center, just below the navel. Exercises can train us to circulate the prana out to other parts of the body.

Prana energy is thought to be what is transferred from your hand to a friend's body when you touch with concern and affection. Raised volume of prana is thought to be the reason why a loving touch feels so much better than a neutral or unfriendly one. In more intense conditions, this positive energy becomes more powerful and, thus, more healing. The laying on of hands is thought to be a transfer of prana current. Both physical and mental energy come from prana. All willpower and all healing arises from control of this energy.

We take in vitality, or prana, from the air as we breathe, and store it in our bodies. Vital prana energy needs to move and be evenly distributed throughout the body to produce health and balance. Hatha yoga teaches control of the prana through physical exercises.

VISHNU MUDRA

Take some air.

Yoga patterns for breathing are designed to help clear your air passages, improve your control and discrimination and bring more prana and oxygen through your body. The Vishnu Mudra position enables you to more easily close alternate nostrils during breathing exercises. Repeat the sequences several times.

SLOW ALTERNATE BREATH

1. Sit comfortably with the tip of your spine on a small pillow. Keep your legs crossed in front of you. Raise your right hand so the palm is toward your face. Specific fingers are used because of their differing magnetic charges. Fold down your index finger and the next finger.

2. Press your thumb to close your right nostril, and inhale with your left nostril to a count of four. Exhale to a count of eight. The exhalation should take twice as long as the inhalation.

3. Now release your thumb and press your left nostril closed with your ring and little fingers as you inhale through your right nostril to a count of four. Then exhale to a count of eight.

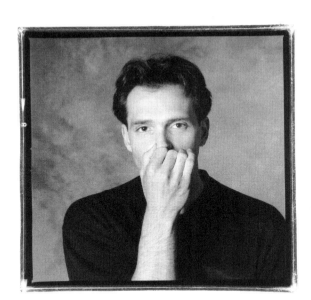
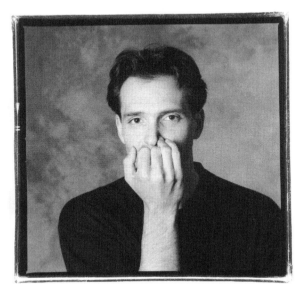

ALTERNATE NOSTRIL BREATH

Switch and sniff.

This breathing pattern helps calm the nerves and improve circulation. It is regarded as a general balancer and purifier of the physical and emotional systems. It is practiced to prepare for more advanced techniques.

1. Close your right nostril with your thumb. Inhale through your left nostril to a count of four.

2. Now pinch your ring and little fingers against your left nostril so both sides are closed. Hold your breath to a count of sixteen.

3. Release your thumb and exhale to a count of eight through your right nostril.

4. Next inhale through your right nostril to a count of four.

5. Pinch both nostrils closed to a count of sixteen.

6. Release your last two fingers so that you can exhale through your left nostril to a count of eight. Repeat the whole cycle several times.

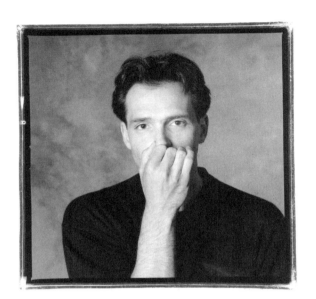
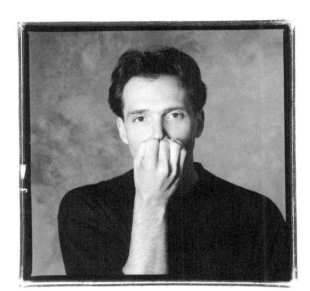
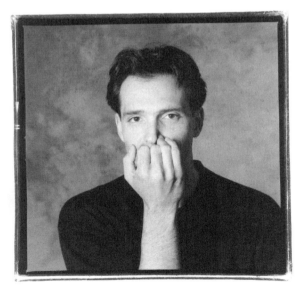

PRANA SEAL

■

Breath envelope.

This posture helps sustain the benefits of your breathing exercises and unites opposing natural energies.

1. Sit in a meditation posture with your legs crossed. Perform your breathing exercises. Afterward, inhale through your nose as you wrap your arms behind your waist. Clasp your right wrist with your left hand.

2. Exhale as you lean your torso forward and relax your neck and forehead toward the floor. Rest in this position for as long as you feel comfortable.

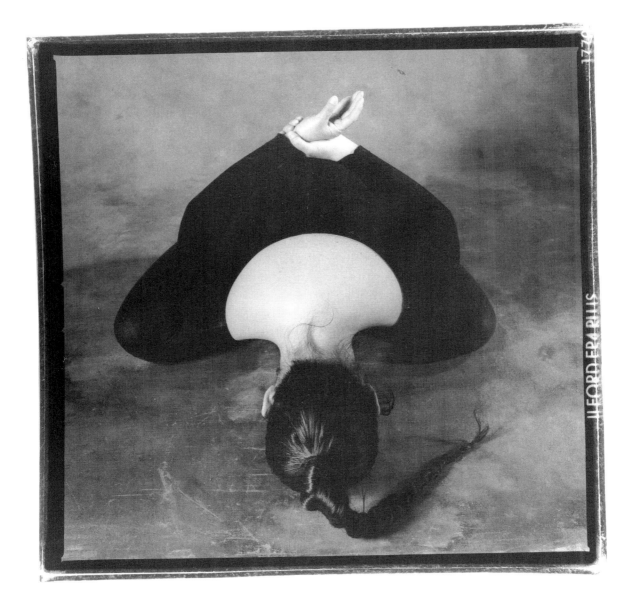

PRANA LOCKS

■■■■■

Keys to air power.

Prana is the spinal energy that moves through the spinal cord and stimulates the various nerve plexus centers. When it rises up to the head, it produces intense states of mental clarity and physical balance. Raising this spine energy, called kundalini, is the aim of prana locks, or bandhas, which close the energy exits for the prana and retain it inside your body. These are part of advanced meditation practice and should be used after much experience with breathing techniques. The ultimate aim of all breathing exercise is to raise the prana energy to the top of the head in order to create mental and spiritual balance.

JALANDHARA BANDHA Press your chin down against your collarbone while you hold your breath. The object of this position is to contain the prana and keep it from leaving your upper body.

UDDIYANA BANDHA Exhale fully and suck in your belly. Pull your abdominal muscles up and back toward your spine. The object of this position is to propel the prana upward through your spine.

MOOLA BANDHA Hold your breath. Contract your buttocks, anal muscles, and abdominal muscles; hold this position. The aim is to contain the lower spine energies within the body and draw them up to unite with the prana currents higher in the spine.

BREATH OF FIRE

███████

Till you're smoking.

This breathing exercise is used on its own or with kundalini poses to trigger circulation and energy flow up the spine toward the brain. When the student learns to stimulate the body's afferent and efferent nerve pulses simultaneously, the nerves send strong currents up the spine. It begins with a warmth in the lower back. This sensation can move up the spine and revitalize you. This is an advanced process, but simple versions of the Breath of Fire can be done effectively. This can be used with the partner poses.

1. Sit upright. Breathe through your nose. As you inhale, puff your abdomen out. As you exhale, contract the abdominal muscles inward sharply. Increase the pace as you go. The breathing becomes deep, rapid, and forceful.

2. Quite the opposite of most yoga breathing patterns, the exhalation is short and hard, while the inhalation is slower and longer in a one to four ratio. Focus your attention on the solar plexus at your diaphragm.

3. After about forty breaths, inhale, apply a prana lock, and hold your breath for a count of forty. When you exhale, do so slowly and evenly. Then begin the rapid Breath of Fire. After several minutes of this pattern, relax, breathe normally and observe your response.

II

THE MOVEMENTS

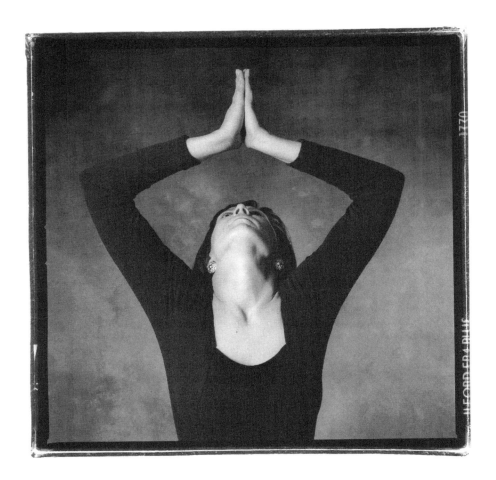

BODY PATTERNS	BACKWARD BENDS
RESTS	TWISTS AND STRETCHES
WARMUPS	BALANCING ACTS
FORWARD MOTIONS	COOLDOWNS

II

THE MOVEMENTS

BODY PATTERNS

Everything ripens and becomes fruit at its hour.
—Divyavadana

Yoga exercises have a sequence that follows the body's natural kinetic patterns. To promote optimum functioning and health, you should exercise one direction of movement and then its opposite. This is the way you move during the Salute to the Sun sequence (page 92). This alternating motion pattern continues throughout the whole yoga workout. It helps to prevent physical strain and to assure balanced muscle development. It also mirrors the pattern of balancing opposites that is at the core of all yoga.

You need not do all the exercises in this book; they are offered for variety and degrees of skill. But always follow your chosen forward stretch with a backward one for balance. Remember to hold the pose for some time. This adds an isometric element that builds strength.

Five-Minute Yoga Bites

Although the full posture cycle done in sequence produces the most dramatic results, short yoga breaks during the day are also extremely beneficial. Just be sure to pair them so you bend both forward and backward. You can also try inserting Rests (page 76) and Balances (page 156) throughout your busy day. Use them as stress reducers, stretch breaks, and brief vacations.

Exercise Cautions

Practice your yoga on an empty stomach, but not if you feel too hungry or dizzy. Drink plenty of water. Work barefoot on a firm mat for cushioning.

A full yoga workout is strenuous. Don't do anything unless it feels completely comfortable, doesn't hurt at all, and causes no strain. Work up slowly to difficult postures. In general, if you have any question, consult your physician for a professional opinion.

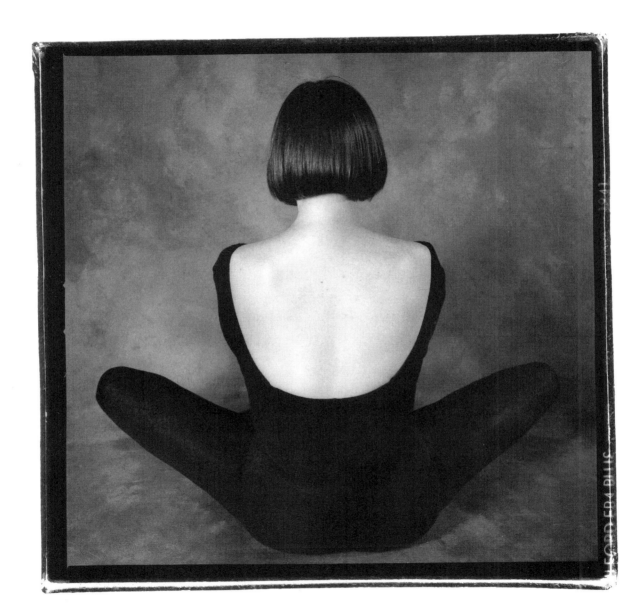

Always warm up, cool down, and do lots of rests in between. Specific exercises can provide extra stress on an injured body part. Don't do headstands and shoulder stands or any exercise that applies pressure to the head if you have: a neck problem, high blood pressure, back pain or injury, or eye problems. Don't do severe back bends if pregnant.

Incorrect forward stretching can aggravate sciatica. Be sure to extend the spine upward and bend at the waist before you stretch forward. Keep knees slightly bent to prevent back aches.

Be careful not to strain your knees by squatting too low or standing too long. If you have recently had an illness or surgery, check with your physician before any exercise.

Otherwise do what feels good and have fun.

OPEN CIRCUITS

Rodney Yee, a San Francisco based yoga instructor, says, "I think of the body as an electrical field that can become overloaded by the intensity of modern life. Clarity comes when we can allow experiences to flow through us rather than to build up pressure and blocks. Yoga strengthens body and mind, enabling us to handle intensity."

Yoga postures are meant to be done gently and held a long time, while you take note of your sensations. Your role is to observe and feel rather than to push yourself. This develops your physical and mental stamina and you can gradually do more and more without strain.

The sequence of enlightenment, or profound understanding, in yoga proceeds from the body to the mind. We build physical strength and agility to engender mental and spiritual flowering. Like gardening, hatha yoga practice can cause strong trees to emerge from delicate seeds.

Not hammer strokes, but dance of the water sings pebbles into perfection.
—Rabindranath Tagore

RESTS

Night falls, and all are dissolved
Into the sleeping germ of life.
—Bhagavad Gita

One thing I've always liked about yoga is that the rests come first, last, and often. But like other aspects of yoga, they differ from ones most of us are familiar with. Unlike rests in other physical exercise, yoga rests are not stops. They are not times to shut off your mind and forget what you are doing. They are not times to flop down and collapse.

Yoga rests are moments for your body to recoup and relax. But they are also periods of continued mental and physical alertness. As in all yoga postures, you take note of your mental and physical states. These are moments for reflection and registering the effects of the movement on your mind and body. Because this attention has no preconceived agenda, content, or judgment, it is very restful. In traditional hatha yoga, you practice a rest, usually Child Pose or Corpse Rest, after each asana.

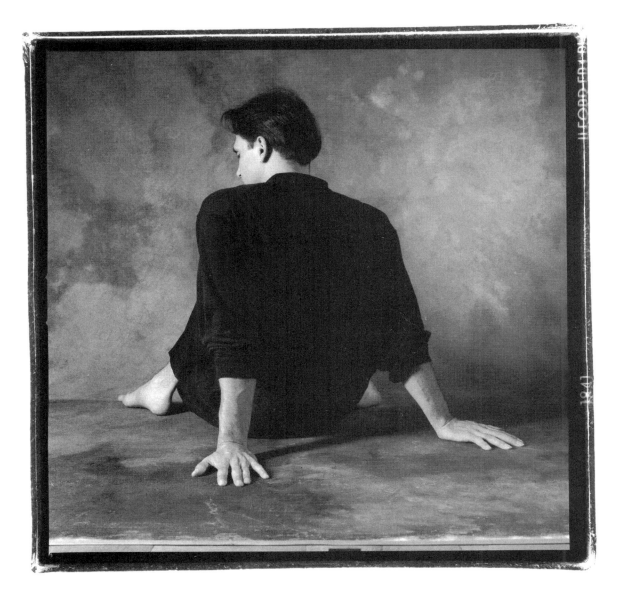

CHILD POSE

■■■■

Baby yourself.

This is a cozy rest that releases tension in your spine and shoulders and that counteracts strain from backward stretches.

1. Kneel and sit on your knees. Exhale as you relax your torso forward to rest on your thighs. Close your eyes.

2. Keep your neck curled forward, chin tucked under, arms relaxed at your sides, palms up. Breathe normally through your nose.

3. Allow your upper back and shoulders to droop more and more toward the floor. When ready, sit up slowly, uncurling your upper back and neck last.

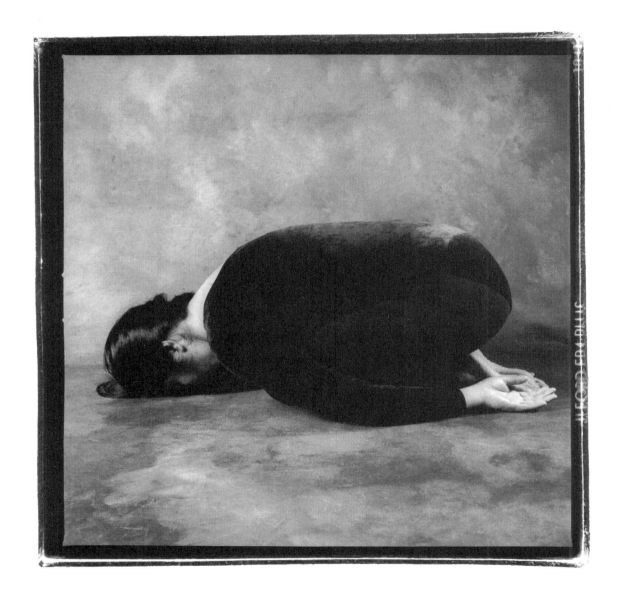

SQUAT REST

Sciatic serenity.

This position opens hip joints to release pressure on the lower back. It relieves pinching of the sciatic nerves leading from the base of the spine across the hips and down the legs.

1. With feet shoulder width apart, bend your knees and squat. Try to keep your heels flat on the floor and parallel rather than turned out.

2. Press your elbows or forearms outward on the insides of your knees so your hip joints are stretched a bit. As you rest, your forehead can lean forward onto your clasped hands.

3. Gradually relax so the position, rather than muscle tension, is holding you in place.

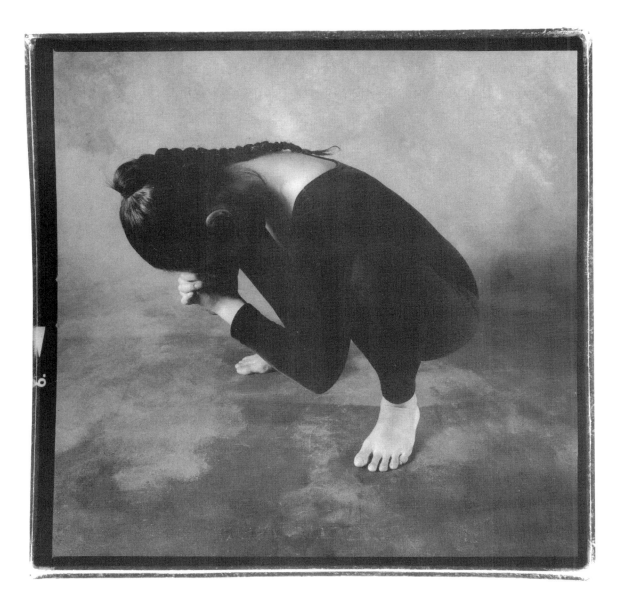

EGG

████████

Coddle yourself.

1. Lie flat and draw both knees over your chest as you exhale.

2. Reach up around your knees so you can cradle them with your arms as you curl your neck forward and your forehead toward your knees.

3. Hold this position and allow the curl stretch to relax your spine and your back muscles. Reverse the movement and unwind slowly.

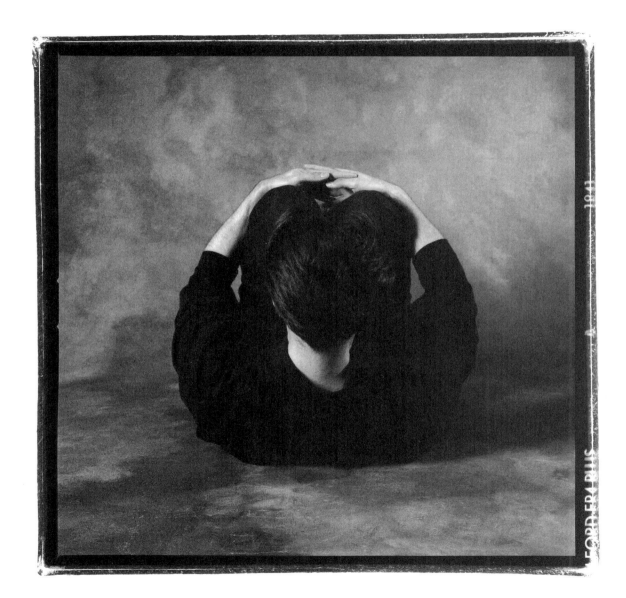

EGG ROLL

Boil.

1. Assume the Egg pose. Increase your armhold on your knees, point your toes, and curl your head firmly toward your knees.

2. Inhale as you rock backward on your spine by tugging your knees a little closer to your chest.

3. As you exhale, push your knees up and away from your torso in order to give your body a forward roll. Slide your palms to your knees if this helps you rock forward.

4. Alternately push and pull so you maintain a rocking motion on your back.

5. When you are through, you can lie flat in the Corpse Rest pose. Or you can increase your rocking and then release your arms as you roll forward, so that you rock onto the soles of your feet and can stand up.

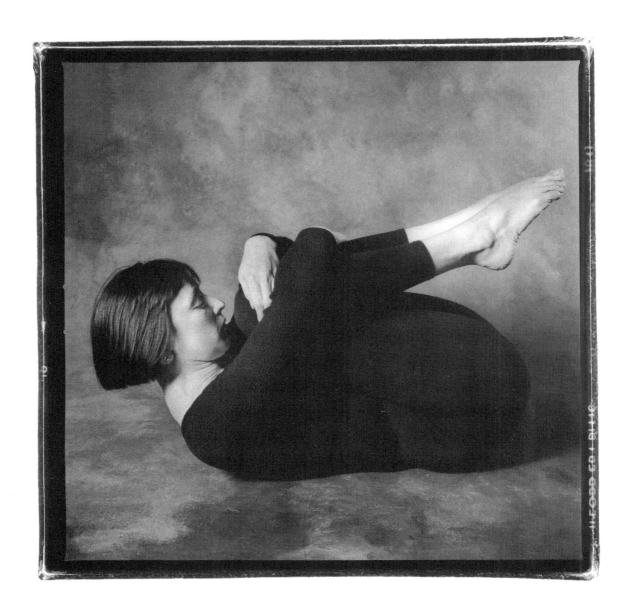

CORPSE REST

████

A drop-dead favorite.

It should be so simple to lie down and relax. However, sometimes we're too tense. If so, the following gentle sequence should do the trick. It can also help you sleep more deeply.

1. Lie down on your back on a flat surface with your arms resting at your sides and your palms up. Try to clear your mind of thoughts other than the feelings in your body. Make a mental note of how your body feels lying on the floor. You can compare this with your sensations at the end of the exercise. Starting with your feet, notice which parts of your body touch the floor and which parts arch away. Do you feel tilted in any direction?

2. Flex and release each joint and muscle working up to the head. Inhale as you flex; exhale as you release. Allow your breathing to massage you from the inside, as though you could exhale through your body and into any tight areas to soften them.

3. If you are still awake when you reach your head, compare how your body feels now to when you started.

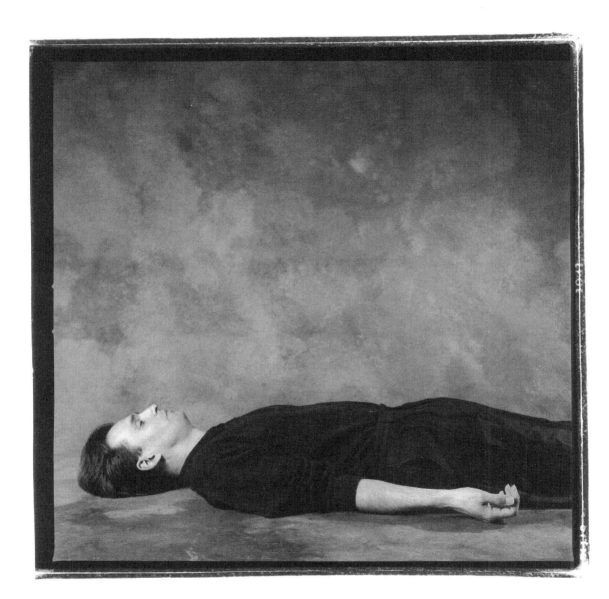

WARMUPS

Day dawns, and all those lives that lay hidden asleep
Come forth and show themselves, mortally manifest.
—*Bhagavad Gita*

Stretching should come only after you warm up. Start very slowly when your muscles are stiff, and increase your pace as you move through the poses. Breathe deeply. Work up to a fast pace so that you are very hot when you reach the last set. It is crucial to remember that any warm up has to make your body actually hot to be effective as a strain preventer.

If you only have time for one asana, the Sun is the one that gives you the most thorough limbering. It can function as an excellent warm up for the full yoga series, and also as a cool down sequence if your practice has been strenuous.

Allow each motion to lead smoothly into the next without a break. Done well, the sequence should feel like a dance. Any day will be brighter following the Salute to the Sun.

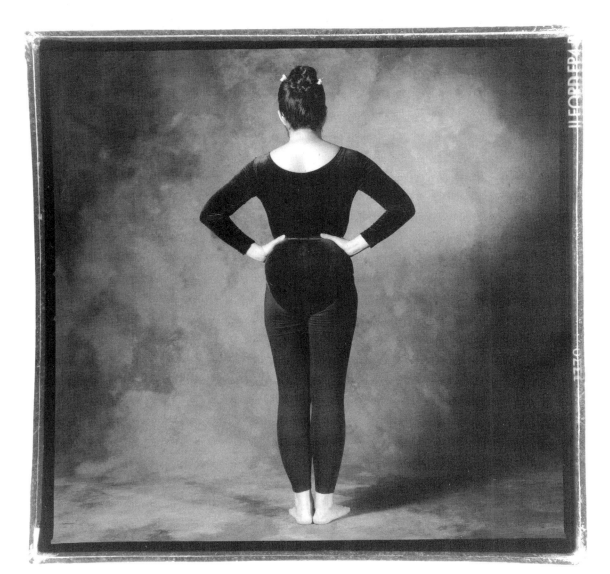

FOURTH CHAKRA STIMULATION

████

Put your heart into it.

Salute to the Sun exercise starts with Heart Chakra Stimulation. But, you can use this on its own or with other poses.

1. Look forward. As you inhale through your nose, draw your hands toward your chest. Keep your palms pressed together, your thumbs and fingers straight.

2. Exhale and firmly press your thumbs and the bones of the heels of your hands against the center chest bone between your ribs.

3. This area on the sternum, or breastbone, is near the location of the solar plexus nerve center known in yoga terminology as the Heart Chakra. Meditation focused here helps stimulate and balance all the functions of the heart.

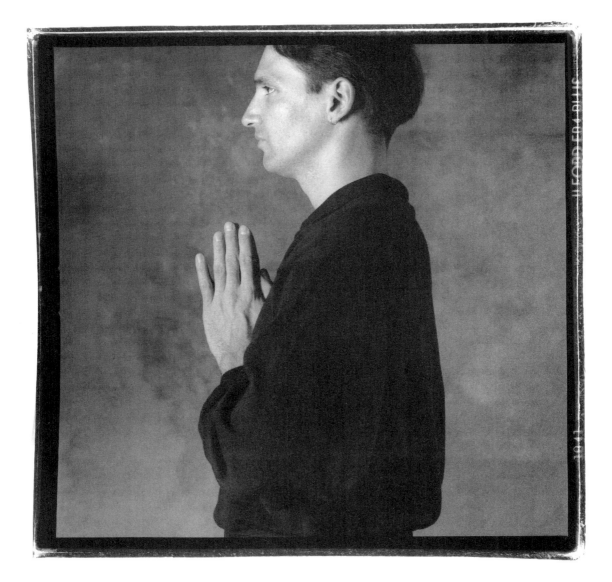

SALUTE TO THE SUN

Start the day relaxed.

A symbol of health and long life, Lord Sun has twelve names and the exercise is done twelve times to honor these powers. The movements stretch the spine in its full range of motion, increase breathing capacity, improve circulation, and limber the arms, legs, muscles, joints, and ligaments.

1. Face the sun. Stand straight with your palms pressed together and your thumbs on the sternum above the solar plexus.

2. Breathe through your nose. Inhale and raise both arms as you arch your torso back.

3. Exhale as you bend forward, drawing your head toward your knees and your hands toward your feet as far as you can.

4. Place your palms on the floor to either side of your feet. Inhale as you tilt your head up, bend one knee and straighten the other leg along the floor behind you.

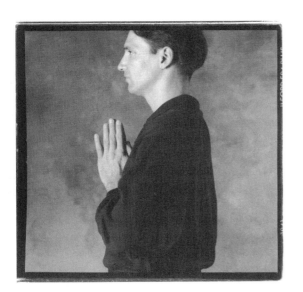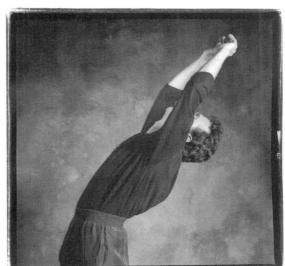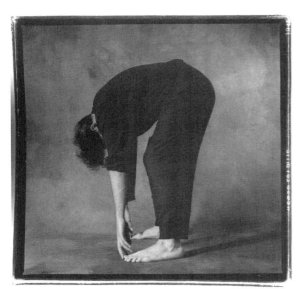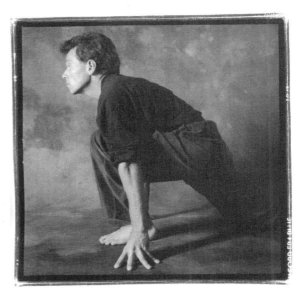

5. Hold your breath as you bring the bent leg back to join the straight one, and try to position your whole body, supported by your arms, in a straight line above the floor.

6. Exhale as you lower your chin, your chest, and your knees to the floor in a snakelike curve.

7. Inhale as you lower your hips toward the floor and arch your spine to raise your torso into the Cobra pose.

8. Exhale as you lower your head and raise your hips so your body forms a triangle, with your knees straight and your feet as flat on the floor as is comfortable.

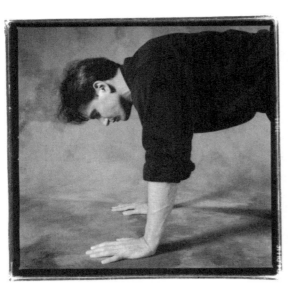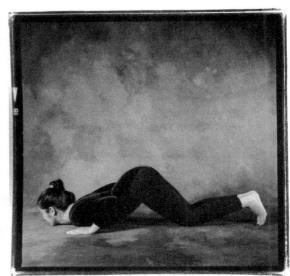

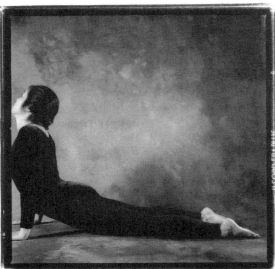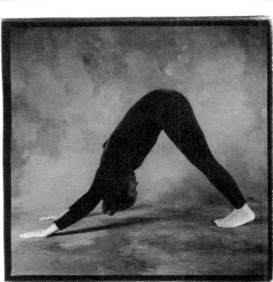

9. Inhale as you begin the return sequence. Lean your body weight forward onto your hands as you drag one leg forward. Bend the knee so you can place the foot flat between your hands if possible. Look up toward the ceiling.

10. Exhale as you bring the second leg forward between your hands. Straighten both knees as you roll your head toward your legs. You can hold your ankles to help the stretch.

11. Inhale, raise your arms, and arch your spine backward.

12. Exhale as you stand straight, bring palms together and press thumbs on sternum Repeat this whole sequence twelve times. As a warmup, the Salute to the Sun sequence should be paced gradually faster, so your circulation improves and your body feels hot and limber for the following exercises.

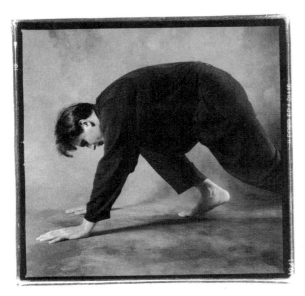 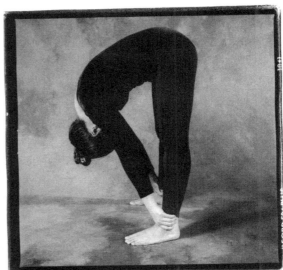

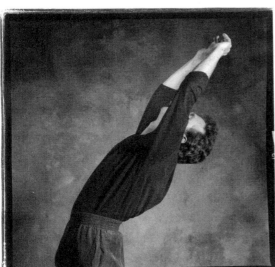 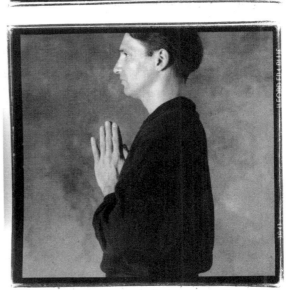

FORWARD MOTIONS

A spirit filled with truth directs its actions to the final goal.
—Mahatma Gandhi

Start your yoga sequence with forward moving exercises. Most people tend to bend in this direction more often during the day than backward and can more easily flex their muscles in this direction. Forward bending postures draw your focus inward and provide a transition into a meditative state.

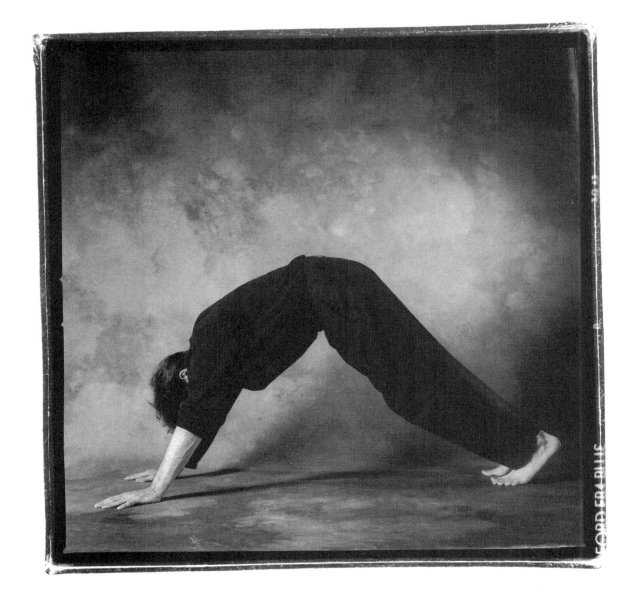

HEADSTAND

▬

Turn your world upside down.

The Headstand pose develops your powers of concentration. Even though this is a relatively difficult posture, it comes at the beginning of the sequence of yoga exercises, because it is so good for circulation to the upper body, especially the brain, and because it releases pressure on the lower back, where most of us are tight. Also keep in mind that it makes no difference whether you can do the whole headstand or not. Try each part and do only what feels comfortable. Next time you'll be able to do more. The Headstand is NOT to be done by persons with a weak neck or with either high or low blood pressure. For variations to increase spine and leg flexibility, try different leg positions, such as Lotus or splits.

1. Kneel. Breathe through your nose. Lean forward at the waist. On a large, flat pillow or mat form a triangle with your elbows and your clasped hands on the floor in front of you.

2. Cradle the back of your head firmly in your palms as the top of your head rests on the mat. With your weight distributed equally between the elbows and hands, almost no weight should remain on your head. This is more a balance exercise than one for strength. Straighten your legs so your body is in a triangle position with your hips up.

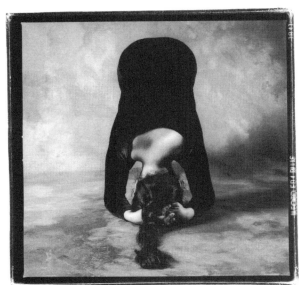
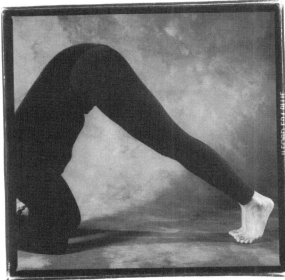

3. Walk forward on your toes so that your spine straightens and your knees come closer to your chest. Then bend your knees as close to your chest as possible. And walk farther.

4. At this point you can push lightly off the floor with your toes and come to a headstand with knees bent. Balance here a while.

5. After this position becomes comfortable, you can slowly straighten your legs to line up with your straight spine. Start with five seconds of balancing on your head. You might work up to several minutes. This is not a position to be held a long time.

6. To come out of the Headstand, bend your knees and lower your legs very slowly. Relax in a kneeling position or Child Pose for a few minutes. Gently roll your head from side to side to relax your neck. Sit upright slowly.

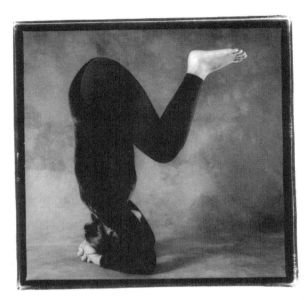
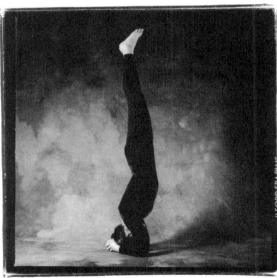

SHOULDER STAND

Sole reversal.

This pose improves circulation to the upper back, brain, thyroid, and parathyroid. It stretches the shoulder muscles and back. Try it for one minute to begin. Work up to no more than fifteen minutes. Breathe normally through the nose. This pose should be followed by the Cow/Cat (pages 124/126) to balance the muscle movement. Do not do the Shoulder Stand pose if you have neck or blood pressure problems.

1. Lie on the floor with your knees bent up over your chest, feet off the floor.

2. Rock your knees and forelegs a bit toward the floor and then quickly back over your chest with enough momentum that your lower back comes off the floor and your knees balance above your shoulders. Place your palms immediately on your lower back for support.

3. Walk your hands toward your shoulders so your back can straighten more. Slowly raise your legs and straighten them above you so your torso and legs form a line. Arch your back and straighten your toes. Relax here for a few minutes.

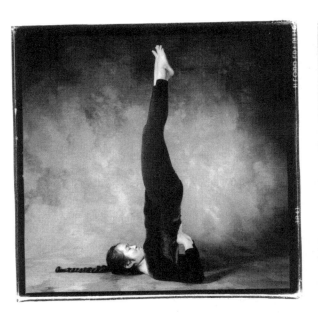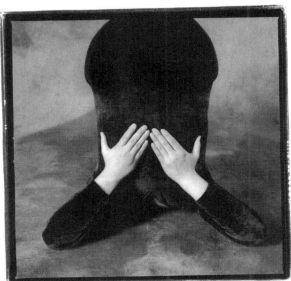

4. A variation requiring excellent balance is done by wrapping one leg around the other as you bend the knees slightly.

5. Come down by reversing the movements. Bend both knees over your head and allow your back to curve slowly forward toward the floor. Lower your palms and legs until you are flat on the floor. Roll your head gently from side to side to relax your neck. Sit up slowly.

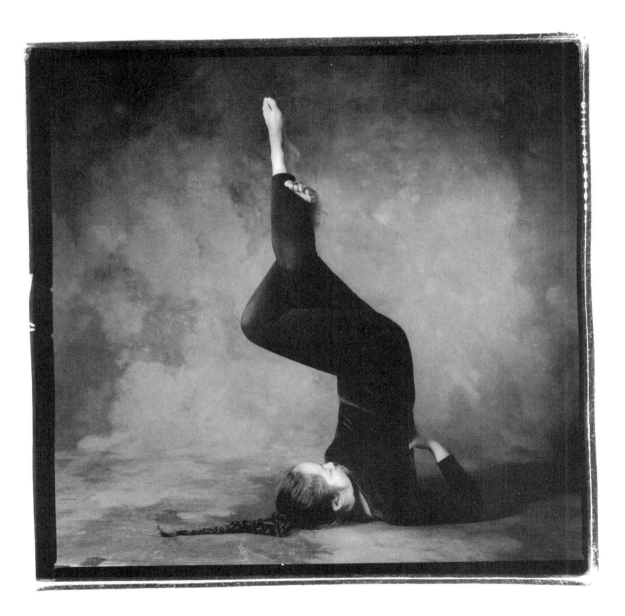

PLOUGH

■■■

Try it in a meadow.

The Plough limbers your entire spine and improves circulation to the upper body. It stimulates the thyroid and various internal organs, while stretching the abdominal muscles. It especially strengthens the cervical region.

1. Lie flat on a mat. Either with your hands supporting your back, as in the Shoulder Stand, or with palms down at your sides, bend your knees and raise your legs and hips, so you can stretch your legs over your head. Your toes will end up touching the floor behind your head. You can also enter this posture from the Shoulder Stand.

2. Now stretch your arms behind your head on the mat, reaching toward your feet. If comfortable, allow your legs to relax and rest your knees on your forehead or on either side of your head.

3. To release the posture, straighten your legs, support your back with your palms and roll your spine and legs back down on the floor. Lie flat a while to relax your muscles. Do the Cobra (page 122) if you feel any muscle cramping.

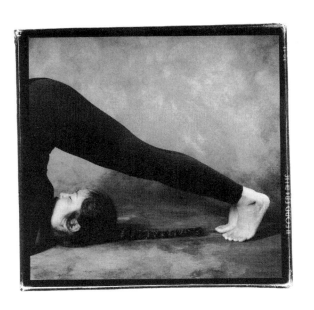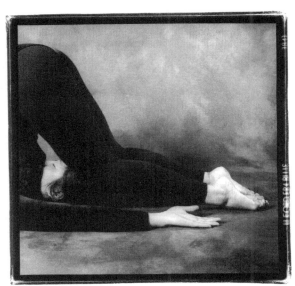

SITTING HEAD TO KNEES

Progress, not perfection.

1. Sit on the floor with legs extended in front of you. Inhale as you raise your arms up above you and straighten your spine. Breathe through your nose.

2. Exhale as you bend at the waist and lean forward over your legs. Reach for your toes. Rest here a while and breathe normally.

3. Your back and leg muscles will become more limber so that you can touch your head to your knees and your fingers can hold your toes. It may seem impossible at first, but gradually it will become easier. Each time, stretch only as far as is comfortable so you do not strain your leg muscles. Keep your knees slightly bent to avoid back strain.

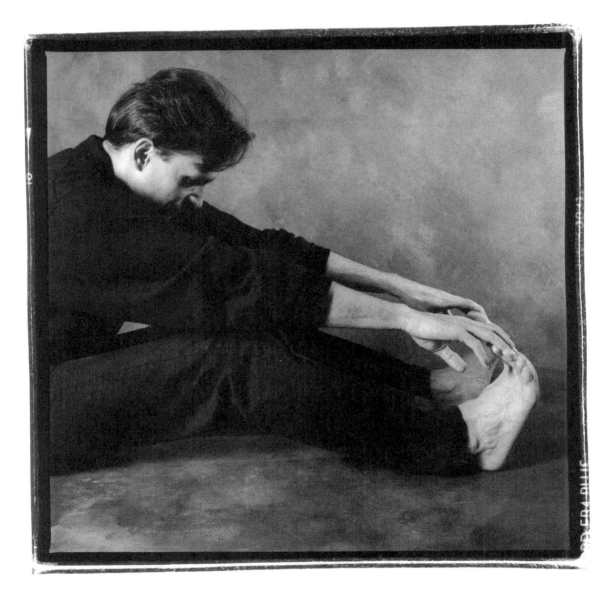

LYING HEAD TO KNEES

Thinking cap tap.

Any version of this pose gives a good stretch to the whole spine. Do as much as you can today and tomorrow your range will be greater.

1. Lie flat on your back. Exhale as you bend one leg and pull it toward your chest. Straighten the other leg on the floor.

2. Simultaneously curve your neck and upper back and draw your forehead toward your bent knee. Rest in this position for a few breaths.

3. Lower your head and leg slowly as you exhale. Repeat the sequence with the other leg.

4. Try lifting both legs at the same time for a double stretch.

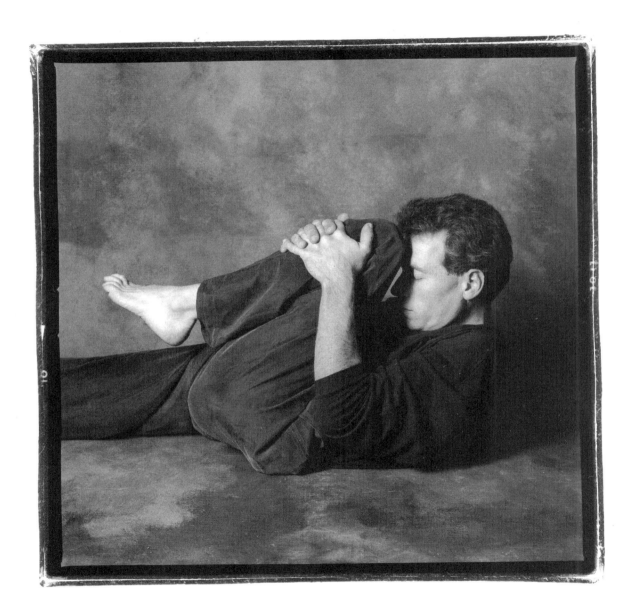

SINGLE LEG RAISE

■

Stretching the point.

This pose stretches the spine and releases tension in the upper and lower back.

1. Lie flat. As you exhale, straighten one knee and draw the leg over your chest with your palms as you bring your forehead or nose toward your knee.

2. Release slowly. Repeat the sequence with the other leg.

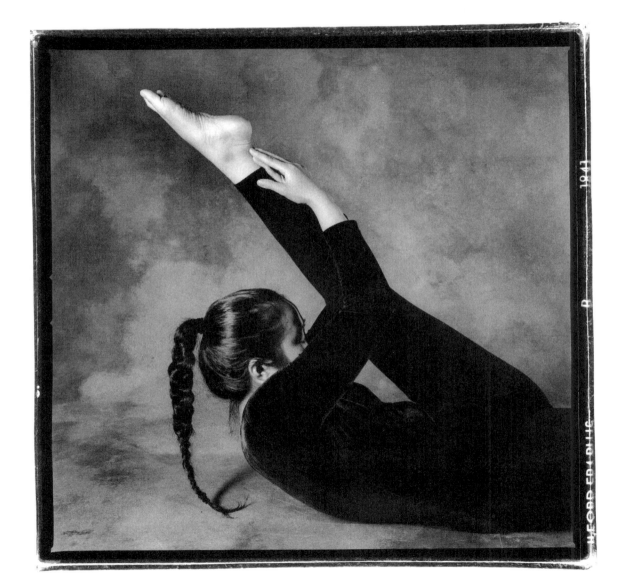

HARE

████████

Jack up your energy.

This movement relieves tiredness, improves circulation, and limbers the joints.

1. From a standing position, exhale and lean forward to grasp your ankles.

2. Look toward the ceiling and inhale through your nose as you squat.

3. Exhale through your nose, contracting your abdomen, as you straighten your knees and bend forward again.

4. Alternate smoothly between the squat and the forward bend. Start slowly and gradually speed up without sacrificing your positions. The breathing becomes deeper and more forceful.

5. When you want to slow down, gradually decrease your leg movement and breathing speeds. End standing up, arms at sides.

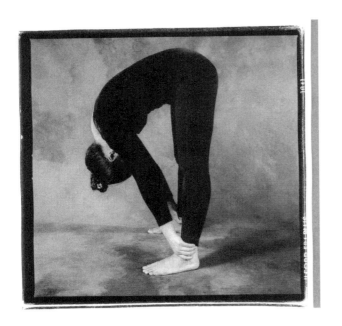 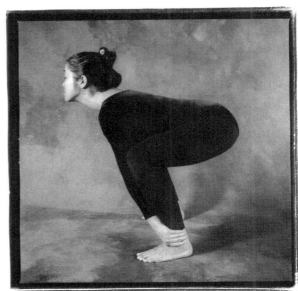

OSTRICH

Look inward.

1. Stand erect and stretch your arms upward. Exhale as you lower your arms and your torso forward.

2. Use your arms to draw your head toward your knees. Inhale. If straight knees are uncomfortable, bend them slightly.

3. Place your palms on or near your feet. Or if you feel quite loose, place your palms on the floor behind your legs.

4. Relax and breathe naturally through your nose.

5. Reverse the sequence and stand up very slowly.

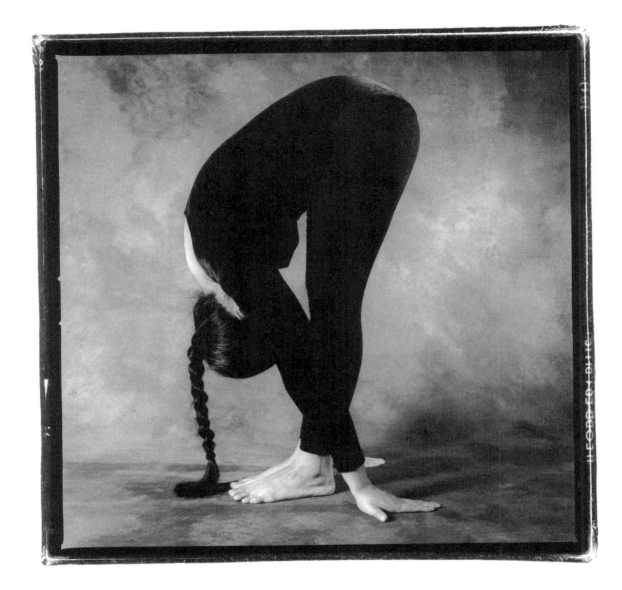

BACKWARD BENDS

The positive always defeats the negative. Courage overcomes fear.
Patience overcomes anger. Love overcomes hatred.
—Swami Sivananda Sarasvati

Backward stretches follow the forward bends. Most of us find these positions slightly more difficult than the forward bends, so it is better to try them when your muscles are fully warmed. These extensions open the chest and, like bending over backward, offer a more expansive, vulnerable mood than the forward foldings.

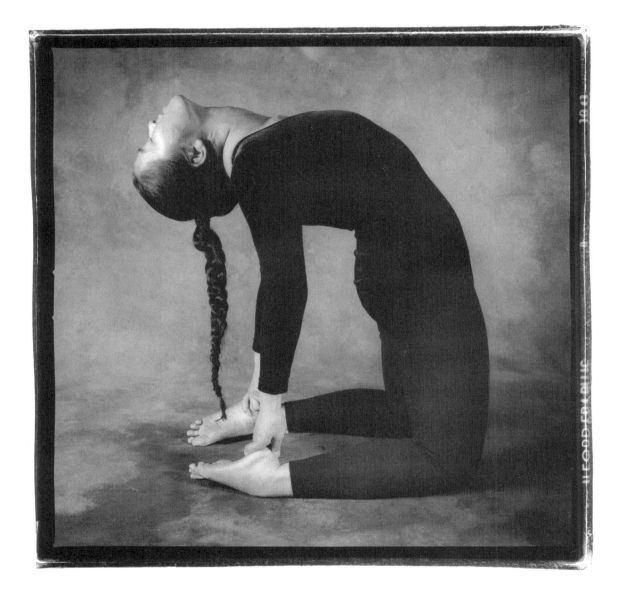

COBRA

████

Curl up for comfort.

This movement strengthens the abdomen and back muscles, particularly the lower back.

1. Lie down flat, face to the floor and rest your forehead on your hands in front of you. Bend your elbows and slide your hands, palms down, to either side of your shoulders. Keep your feet together and your elbows close to your sides.

2. Inhale through your nose as you roll your head and neck back and up so you can look toward the ceiling. Keep your shoulders low and relaxed as you begin to raise your chest off the floor. Try to use your arms as little as possible so the muscles working are mainly in your back and abdomen.

3. Arch your spine backward as far as is comfortable while keeping your abdomen on the floor as much as possible. Hold this position a while.

4. Reverse the process as you unroll, until you are lying down again.

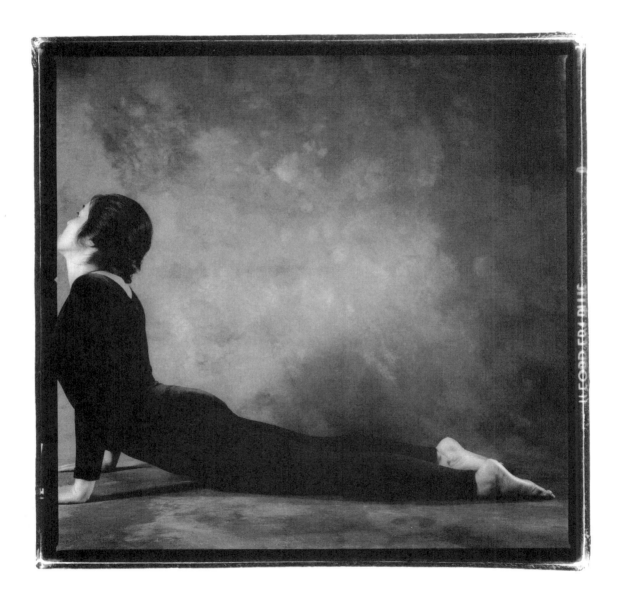

COW

Bovine bend.

When on your hands and knees, you can feel that your spine is relieved of the usual downward pressures from sitting and standing that can cause lower back pain. Done regularly this sequence can prevent and relieve most lower back aches.

1. Begin on your hands and knees, with your knees about hip width apart for balance.

2. As you inhale, tilt your head back and look up at the ceiling.

3. Simultaneously allow your waist to drop and your hips to tilt up, so your spine has a deep bend.

4. Slink directly into the Cat position which follows.

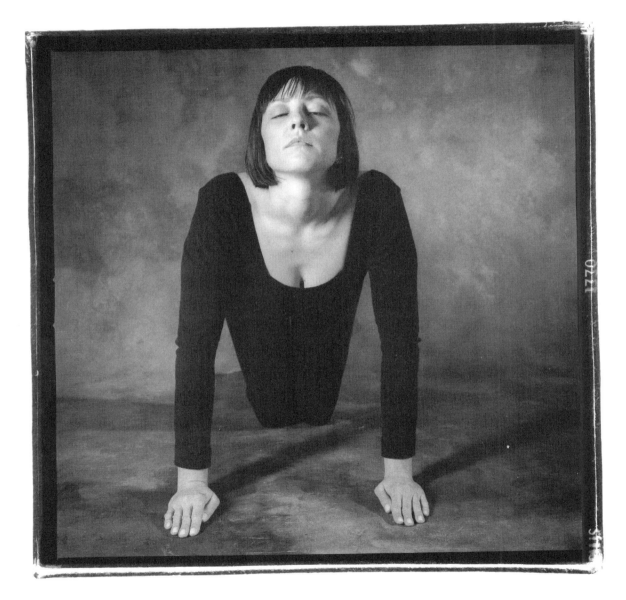

CAT

Feline stretch.

1. Starting from the conclusion of the Cow pose, exhale as you lower your head, drawing your chin toward your chest.

2. At the same time, tuck under your pelvis and arch your back toward the ceiling.

3. Alternate Cow and Cat positions with each long inhalation and exhalation. Allow the motion to be continuous, slow and smooth.

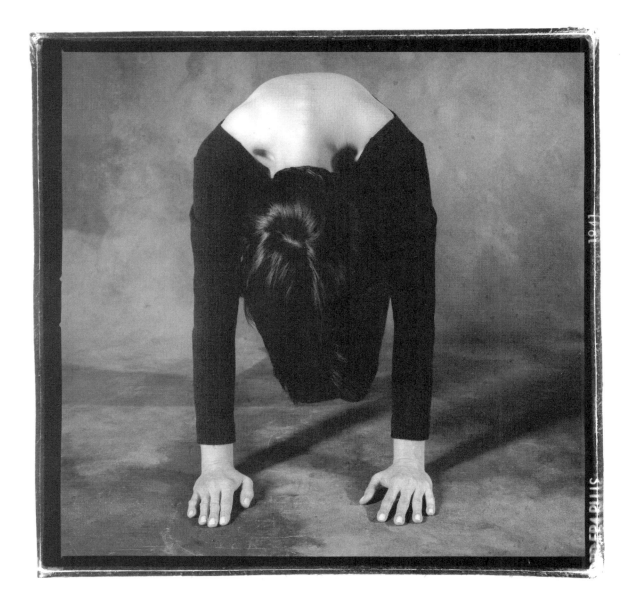

CAT STRETCH

Keeps your spine purring.

1. On your hands and knees, inhale through your mouth, and look up at the ceiling. At the same time, stretch one leg out and up behind you and drop your spine.

2. Exhale as you curl your neck forward and arch your back upward. Bend your extended knee and draw it under your chest as close to your chin as is comfortable.

3. Alternate these movements as you breathe, allowing the sequence to become smooth and dancelike.

4. Switch to the other knee and try the movement with the opposite leg.

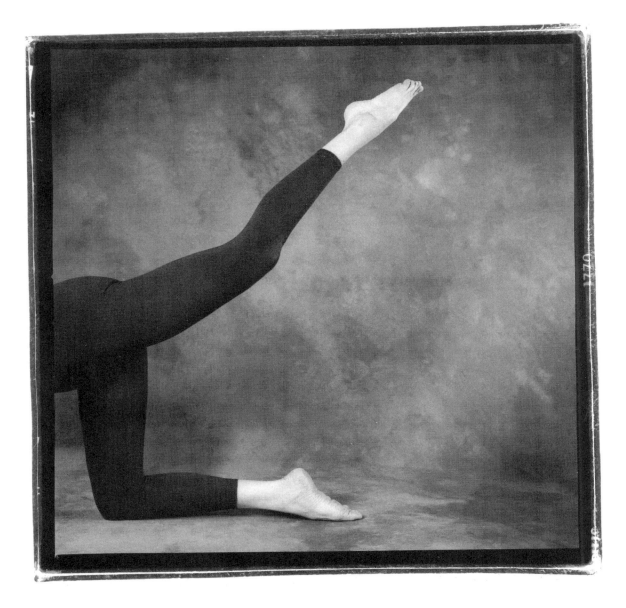

MINNOW

Little muscle movements.

This stretch is a good preparation for the Fish and other postures requiring limber neck and shoulders. It relieves upper back tension when few other moves reach the area between your shoulder blades.

1. From a sitting position, curl down onto your back, drawing your knees over your chest and supporting your torso on your elbows.

2. Draw your knees closer to your chest as you arch your neck and head back. Keep your weight supported on your elbows so your back and shoulders can be loose.

3. Allow your shoulders and neck to relax so your head can drop as low to the floor behind you as possible. Don't stretch your chest up as you drop your head back. Turn your head from one side to the other, trying to touch your chin to either shoulder.

4. Next, let your head rest in the center and shift your weight from one elbow to another to help release your shoulder muscles.

5. Slowly raise your head, roll forward, and sit up.

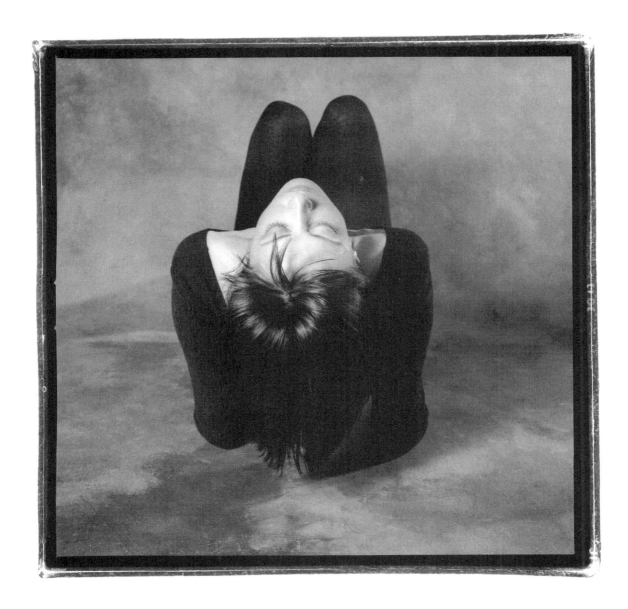

FISH

▆▆▆▆▆

Gotta stretch.

This exercise is a deeply relaxing stretch for the cervical and lumbar regions and for the shoulders. This pose improves circulation to these areas and strengthens the thyroid and parathyroid. Breathe deeply through your nose to help relieve asthma or bronchial stress.

1. Either sit on the floor, with your legs loosely crossed, or kneel, with your legs tucked under you whichever is comfortable. Different leg muscles will be toned. Lean back onto your forearms. Allow your weight to rest on your elbows as you arch your head and neck backward.

2. Slowly slide your elbows out from under you until the tip top (not back) of your head is resting on the floor and your back is arched. Your arms are now free either to rest at your sides or to be raised over your head to stretch your legs and chest even more.

3. Inhale through your nose as you lift your arms above your head. Lie down flat for a fuller stretch. Exhale as you bring your arms back to your sides. Alternate arm positions with your breathing.

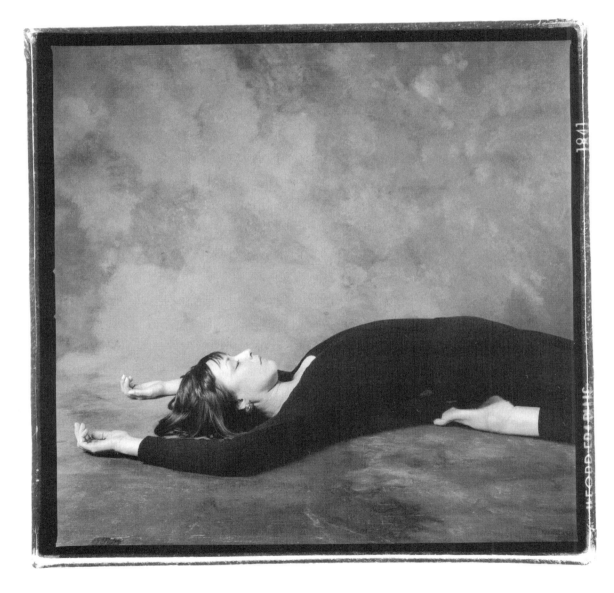

CAMEL

████████

Oasis for the spine.

1. Kneel and sit on your heels. Inhale as you raise your thighs and torso straight up over your knees. Allow your neck to arch back as you grasp your heels with your hands.

2. Exhale as you arch your back and neck more to increase the stretch. Hold this pose and breathe normally through your nose.

3. To unwind, exhale as you lower your chin, straighten your back, and sit down on your shins.

4. Rest your back by leaning your torso forward onto your thighs and relaxing your arms beside your legs, as in the Child Pose.

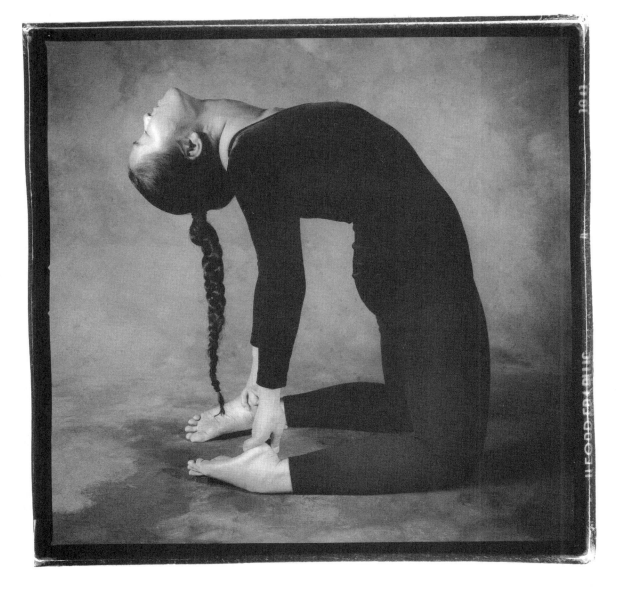

BOW

___

Body archery.

1. Lie flat with your forehead on the floor. Bend your knees and reach behind you to grasp both ankles.

2. With arms straight, inhale and raise your head, chest, and legs to form a backward arch with your whole body. The stretch comes from trying to straighten your legs and torso while still clasping your ankles.

3. Breathe normally and hold the pose for up to thirty seconds. Exhale as you slowly release the pose and lie down.

4. A variation for more stretch is to inhale and rock back, then exhale and rock forward as you hold your ankles.

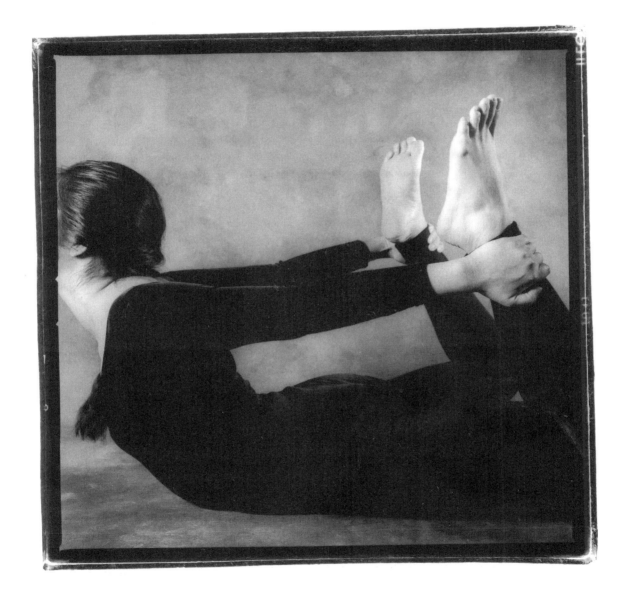

WHEEL

■■■■

Well rounded.

This pose tones muscles and ligaments of the legs, hips, shoulders, arms, and spine. It counteracts a forward hunch in your posture.

1. Lie down on your back with your knees bent and your feet on the floor, heels drawn up toward your buttocks.

2. Reach your arms above your head and place your palms on the floor, fingers pointing to your feet.

3. Push with your arms and legs so your body arches up off the floor. Breathe through the nose. Arch a bit more.

4. Now gradually lower your body to the floor and slowly straighten out.

5. A variation is to arch your neck and lower your chin and elbows toward the floor when in the full Wheel for a longer stretch. You can also walk your hands and feet closer toward each other as you become more comfortable.

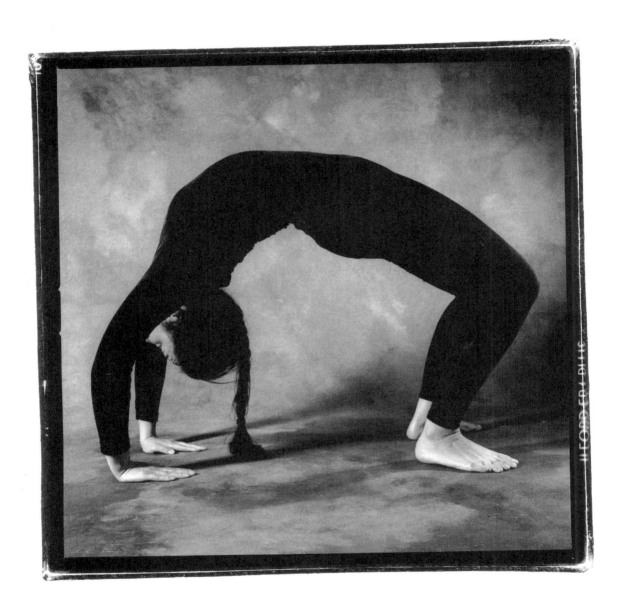

TWISTS AND STRETCHES

*A thousand reasons for worry, a thousand reasons for anxiety oppress
day after day the fool, but not the wise man.*
—*Hitopadesa of Narayana*

To thoroughly limber and strengthen all the muscles and joints
of the body, sideways and circular moves that ensure full range of
motion are included in the yoga workout.

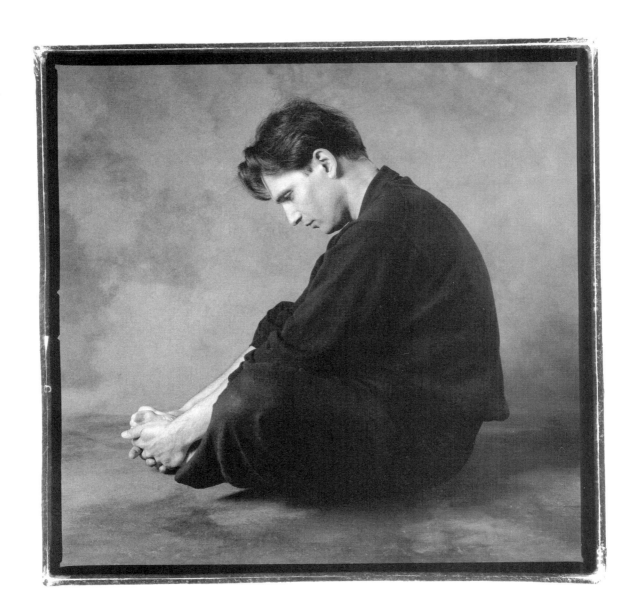

NECK ROLLS

Helps keep them away.

This movement tones neck muscles and frees neck motion.

1. Sit with your spine erect, shoulders relaxed and arms resting in your lap.

2. Slowly roll your head to one side; then down to the front; then to the other side; then backward. Allow the roll to be smooth and continuous.

3. Repeat the sequence several times. Notice where your motion catches.

4. Then reverse the direction, and roll your head to the other side.

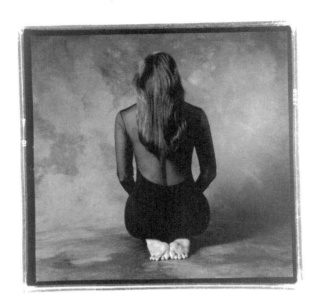

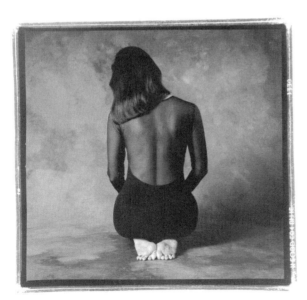

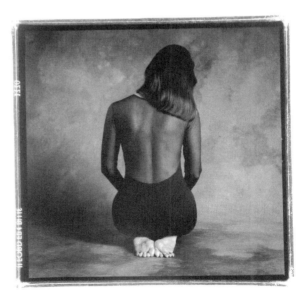

WARRIOR

█████

Shoulder guard.

1. Sit with your legs stretched out straight. Bend one leg so that the knee is bent on the floor and the heel rests under the opposite hip. Raise and bend straight leg, placing knee on top of the first and the foot positioned outside its opposite hip. Your legs will form a triangle in front of you, with your knees together at the apex.

2. Straighten your spine, look forward, and stretch your arms as follows: Clasp hands behind you with one elbow up and the other bent behind your back. Just touch fingertips, if you cannot hold hands.

3. Relax a while. Then switch arm positions to limber the other shoulder.

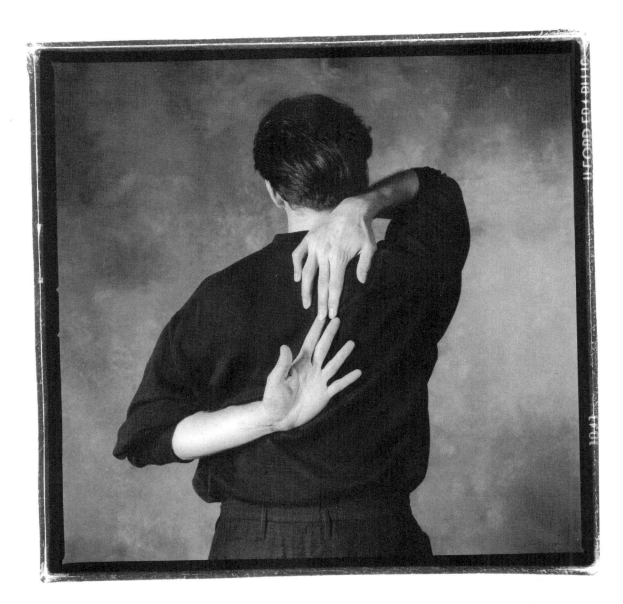

COW'S HEAD

■

Hand-in-hand flexibility.

To release tense muscles between the shoulder blades, this posture is a valuable stretch for a neglected area. The pose develops the trapezoid muscles at the top of the shoulders, opens the rib cage, and helps prevent calcium deposits in the arm joints.

1. Sit with knees bent on the floor. Slide your heels to the outside of their respective hip joints, so the toes point away from the body. This requires such flexibility that few people should do it right away. A simple variation is to kneel and sit on your heels. Raise one arm over your head. Bend the elbow. Place the palm on the back of your neck.

2. Now bend your other arm behind you near your waist and place your hand palm out on your upper back near your shoulder blades. Straighten your back. Reach your hands toward each other until you can touch fingers. Go farther each time until you can clasp hands. Repeat the sequence on the other side. One side will be noticeably easier to stretch than the other.

3. If comfortable, lean your torso forward until you touch the floor with your forehead. Sit up and release the pose slowly.

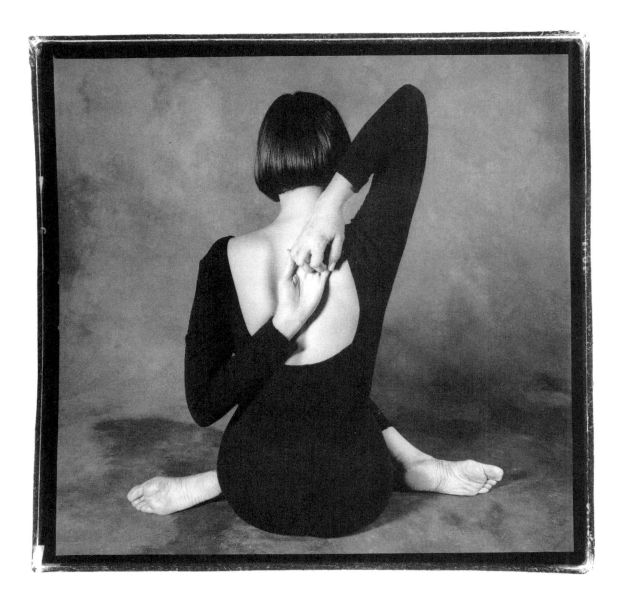

LEG JOINTS OPENER

Very hip.

This posture can help relax the hip joints before meditation. It also loosens the knees and thighs before leg exercises. Do not press your joints beyond a comfortable stretch or you can strain the muscles and ligaments.

1. Sit comfortably with knees bent and legs crossed at the ankles. Then uncross your ankles and place the soles of your feet together; hold your toes with clasped hands. Use the grasp of your feet to help you keep your spine straight.

2. Exhale as you lightly press your knees out and down toward the floor. Inhale as you draw them up toward the ceiling.

3. Start slowly and move more quickly as you feel comfortable.

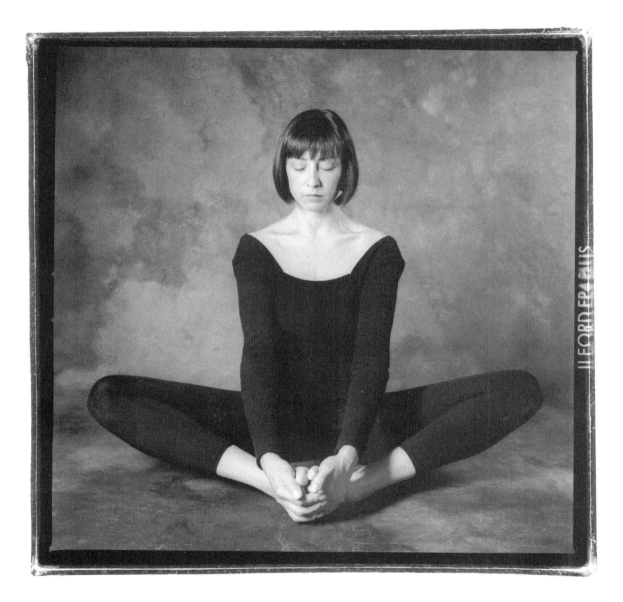

SPINE TWIST

Look back in repose.

1. Sit on the floor with your knees drawn up and bent in front of your chest and feet flat on the floor. Now allow your left knee to relax outward and draw the heel toward the crotch, allowing your knee to rest on the floor.

2. Cross your right foot over the left knee so it rests flat to the left side of the left knee. Slide your left foot to the outside of your right hip.

3. With the left hand, grasp the arch of the left foot. Do this either by placing the arm on the right or left side of the right knee, whichever is comfortable.

4. Now look to your right and behind you as you wrap your right arm behind your back, or rest it on the floor for support.

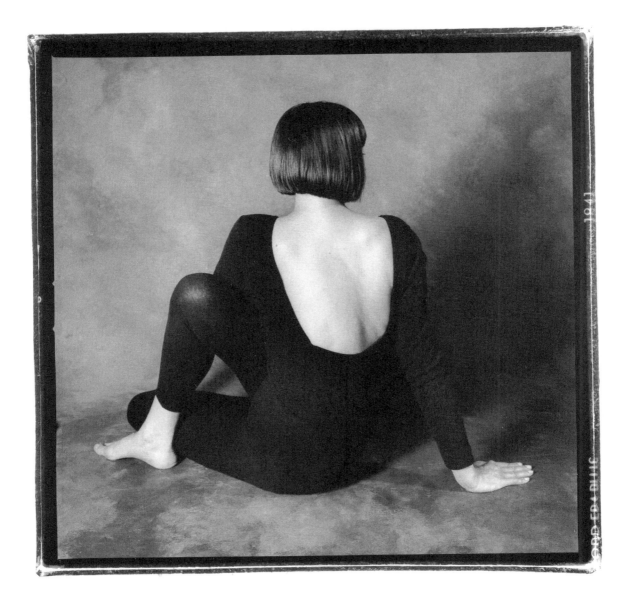

5. With your right arm reach behind you toward either your right thigh or hip. Hold your chest erect. Use the leverage of the position to twist your spine backward.

6. Slowly unwind one limb at a time. Repeat this sequence with the reverse arm and leg. Any approximate position of this asana is good for the spine. You will gradually be able to twist all the way back.

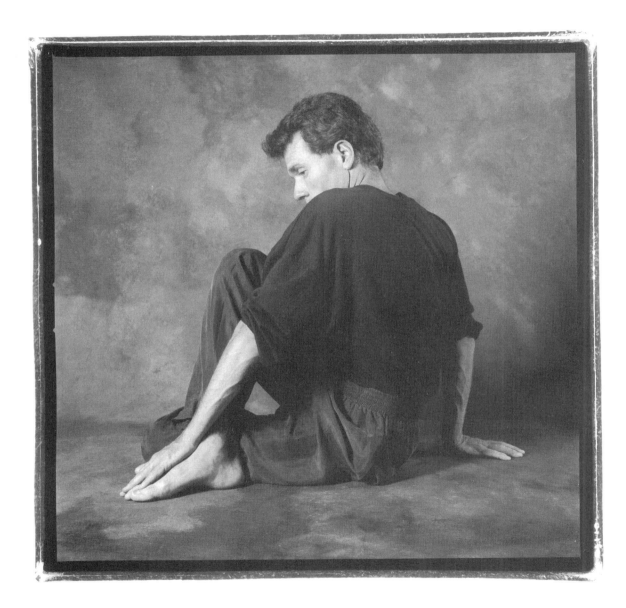

TRIANGLE

A sideways perspective.

This pose stretches your trunk muscles and spine. It improves flexibility of the hips, legs and shoulders.

1. Stand straight, arms at your sides, palms on outer thighs, feet just more than shoulder width apart. A wider placement gives less stretch to your waist, but may be more comfortable.

2. Inhale and raise one arm to the side, palm facing front.

3. Keeping your knees straight, exhale as you bend to the side over your lowered arm and stretch your upper arm to the side above your head, parallel to the floor. Your head stays in a straight line with your spine, almost parallel to the floor, face forward.

4. Slide your lower hand toward your ankle. Be careful to bend sideways rather than forward. Hold this pose from a few seconds to a few minutes. Breathe through your nose.

5. Inhale as you straighten up slowly. Then try the pose to the opposite side.

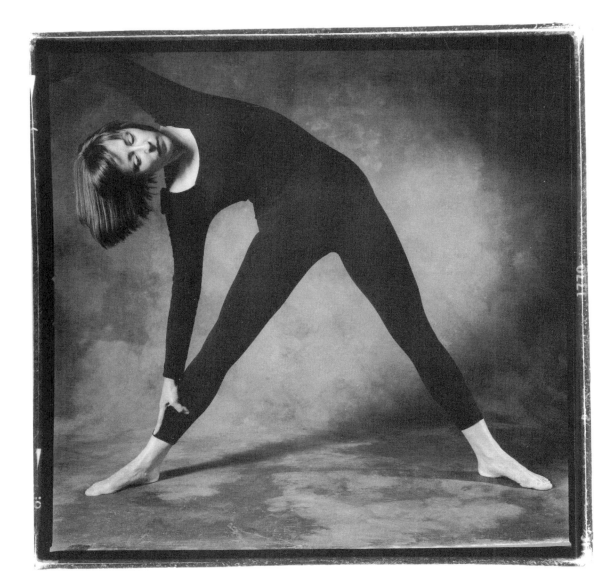

BALANCING ACTS

A pure and strong will is all powerful.
—Vivekananda, c. 1890

Good balance is a crucial part of any physical agility. Yoga balance poses include the aspect of mental balancing as well. Assuming a pose and then maintaining a meditative state increases your mental relaxation, clarity, sense of wellbeing and ability to focus.

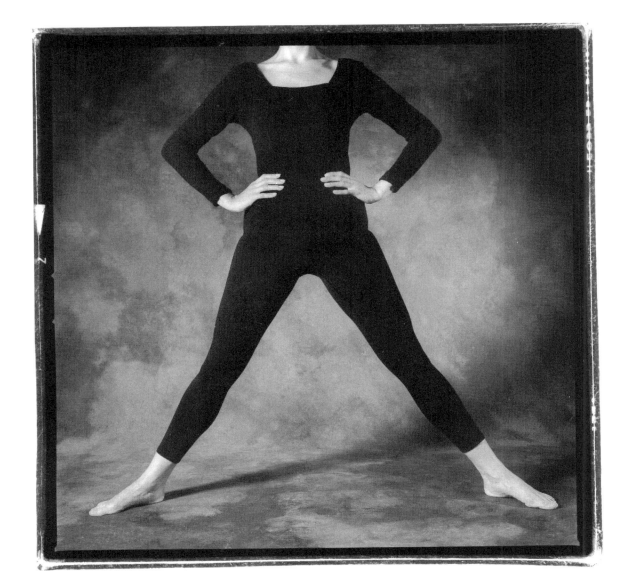

DANCER

Feel the music.

This pose develops balance and concentration. It stretches the leg muscles and joints and tones the arms.

1. Squat while balancing on your toes. You can start with your hands on your hips.

2. Focus your sight on a point in front of you at eye level. Relax your breathing in your abdomen. Inhale as you spread your arms to either side and over your head. When your palms meet, center them over your head.

3. Straighten your back and relax in this position as long as is comfortable, keeping your eye position steady for balance, even if you close your eyes.

4. Slowly unfold. Sit down and make circles with your ankles to relax the joints.

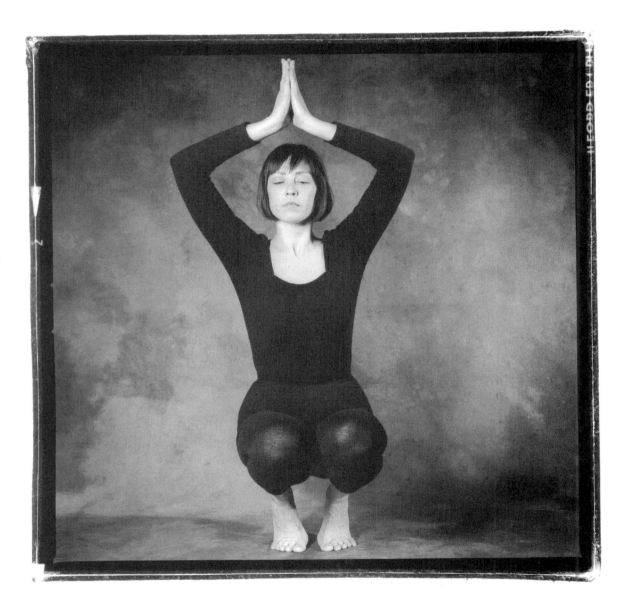

HALF BEAR

Ursa Minor.

This pose improves balance and concentration as it stretches the inner thigh muscles and hamstrings.

1. Sit on the floor with a straight back, your knees bent outward and the soles of your feet touching. Grasp the toes of one foot with the hand on the same side.

2. Inhale as you roll your weight backward a bit onto your tailbone. Straighten your leg out to the side. Hold the toes firmly to improve balance.

3. Exhale as you fold your arm and leg down again. Now try this with the other leg.

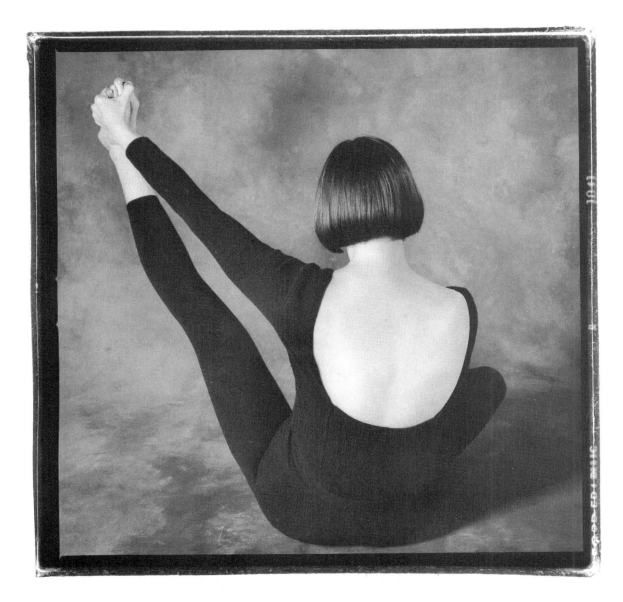

FULL BEAR

██████

Ursa Major.

To improve your balance, focus your sight on a central point in front of you at eye level. Hold this point of concentration throughout the pose. When the Half Bear is comfortable, try the exercise with both legs at once.

1. Start with your legs bent and the soles of your feet touching so you can firmly grasp the toes of each foot with your hands.

2. Roll back to balance on your hips so your feet are off the floor.

3. Inhale as you stretch your arms and legs out to the sides. Gradually straighten your legs as much as is comfortable.

4. Balance in this position for a minute or two, breathing normally.

5. Reverse the motion by bending your legs and arms slowly to resume your original sitting position.

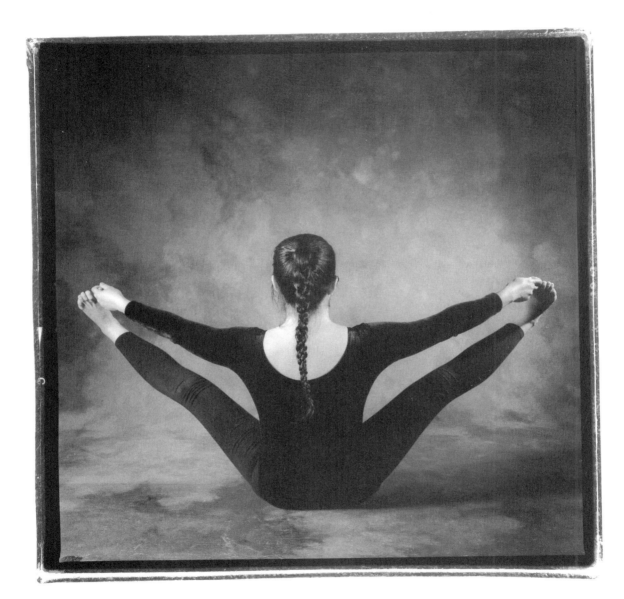

CROW

—

. . . If you can do it.

1. Squat with your feet and knees wide apart and your arms between your knees. Your fingers are spread, palms flat on the floor. Rest on the balls of your feet.

2. Bend your elbows as you turn them outward and your palms inward, fingers toward each other. Focus your sight on a point on the floor a few feet in front of you. Keep this sight point throughout the pose. (If you look directly down, you will tend to fall forward.)

3. Roll your weight forward onto your arms and wrists. When you feel you can roll no further, raise your feet off the ground and roll forward more until your body weight is all on your arms. Keeping your chin up and your eyes focused in front of you is vital to the balance.

4. Relax here for up to a minute. Come down slowly feet first. Then sit down and relax your arms.

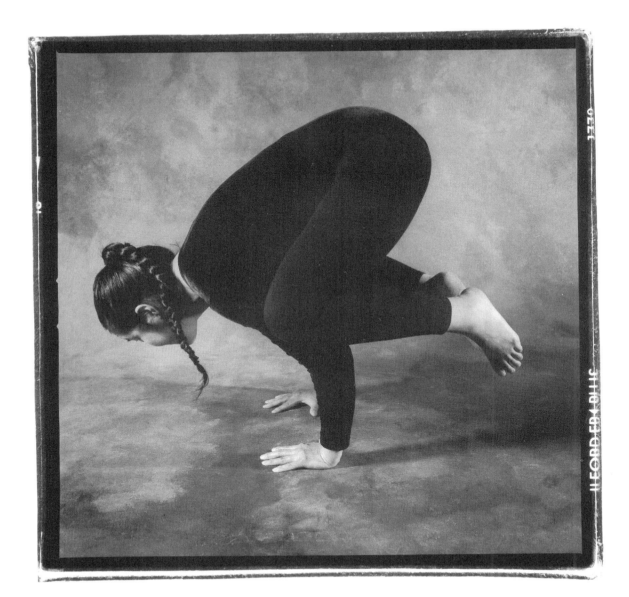

TREE

■

Branch out.

This pose improves balance and circulation as it limbers leg and arm joints.

1. Stand straight and focus your eyes on a spot in front of you at eye level. Keeping this visual focus steady throughout the exercise is key to keeping your balance. Move slowly.

2. Shift your weight to one foot. Bend the other knee to the side and place the foot as high as is comfortable on the inside of the other thigh.

3. Stretch your bent knee out so that your bent leg is almost at right angles to the standing one.

4. Balance for a while with your hands on your hips. Then try raising both arms straight over your head until your palms touch and form a pyramid as in the Dancer pose.

5. Release the posture as slowly as you began it. Try with the other leg.

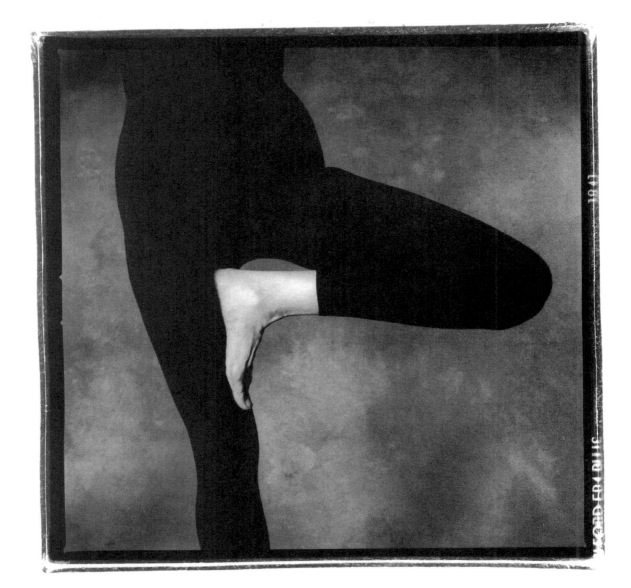

EAGLE

Nest rest.

The Eagle improves your balance and stretches upper back muscles and hip and knee joints.

1. Stand straight and focus your sight on one spot in front of you at about eye level. Shift your weight onto one leg. With knee bent, raise the other leg off the ground. Bend the standing knee slightly.

2. Wrap the raised leg around the front of the standing leg and tuck the raised foot behind the other knee. To balance comfortably you may need to bend the standing knee more.

3. Now follow suit with your arms. Wrap the arm on the folded leg side around the other arm so they cross over at the elbow and wrist and you can clasp your hands palm to palm. You'll need to bend your elbows a lot.

4. Place your forehead on your clasped hands and rest in this pose as long as is comfortable. Release the pose slowly. Repeat on other leg.

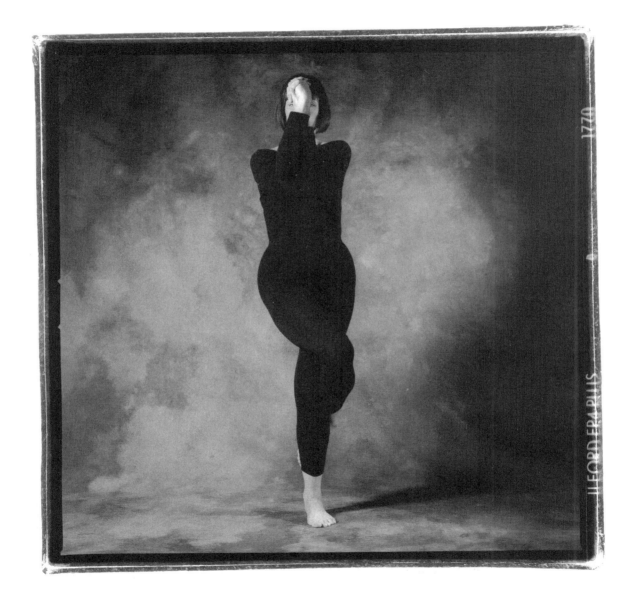

LORD NATARAJA POSE

████

The mythic first yoga teacher.

1. Standing as erect as is comfortable, find your balance on one leg. Maintain your balance by keeping your eyes fixed on one spot straight ahead.

2. Reach behind you and grab the foot of the free leg. Extend the leg and arch your back. Straighten the free arm in front of you parallel to the floor. Balance a while.

3. Release the pose slowly. Repeat the sequence with the other leg.

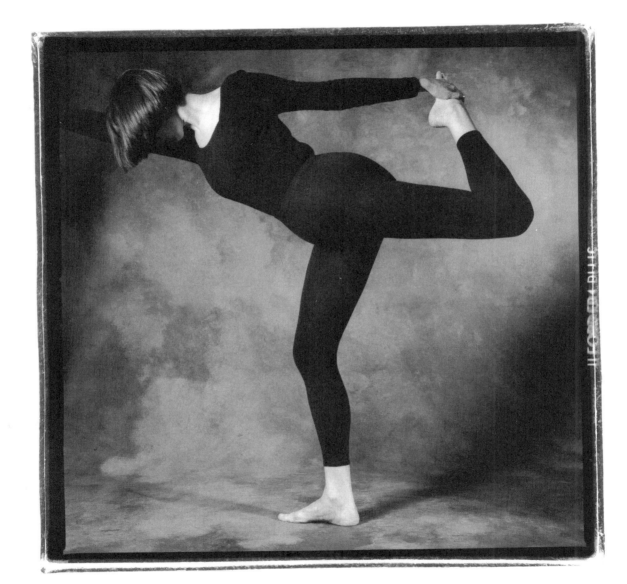

STANDING HALF LOTUS

███████

Bound for balance.

1. Stand up straight and focus your sight on one central spot in front of you at eye level. Shift your weight onto one leg. Bend the other knee to the side and use your hand to lift the foot to rest on the opposite thigh.

2. Let go of the foot. Now wrap the same side arm behind your back so that your fingers can grasp the upturned toes. If this is not comfortable, simply rest your arm behind you. Next, fold your other arm behind you. Balance a few moments.

3. A variation is to exhale as you bend your torso forward slowly and draw your head toward your knees. Resting your free hand on the ground for balance helps make this a comfortable pose.

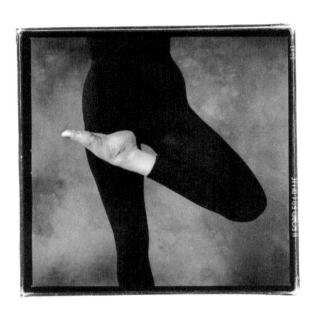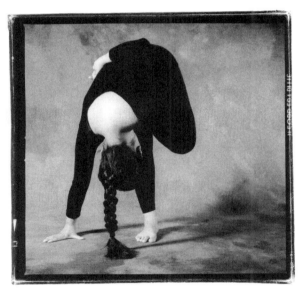

COOLDOWNS

It may take a little selfdiscipline, but be simple, be kind.
—Maharishi, ***Unconditional Life***

Cooling your muscles after a strenuous workout is as important as warming them beforehand. Gradual change is easier on the body than sudden shifts. Warmups and cooldowns help prevent strain. Traditional yoga sequencing, with a rest pose between each posture, takes care of this risk of injury. And most people enjoy ending their sequence with a final rest phase, no matter how many rests came earlier. However, if you choose to speed up your workout and do not rest between the poses, then you do need to practice cooldown postures as the finale to your session.

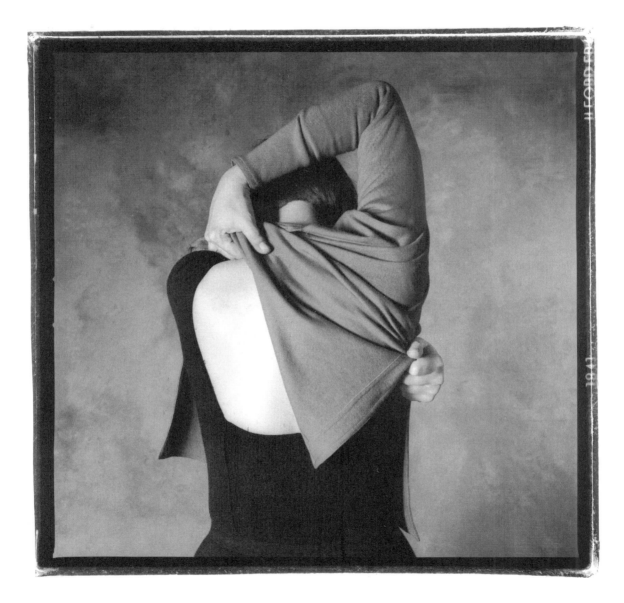

SALUTE TO THE SETTING SUN

Go through the complete Salute to the Sun sequence as described at the beginning of the Warmups section twelve times (see page 92). Start at a brisk pace and gradually lessen your pace. As you finish, you should feel as though you are dancing in slow motion.

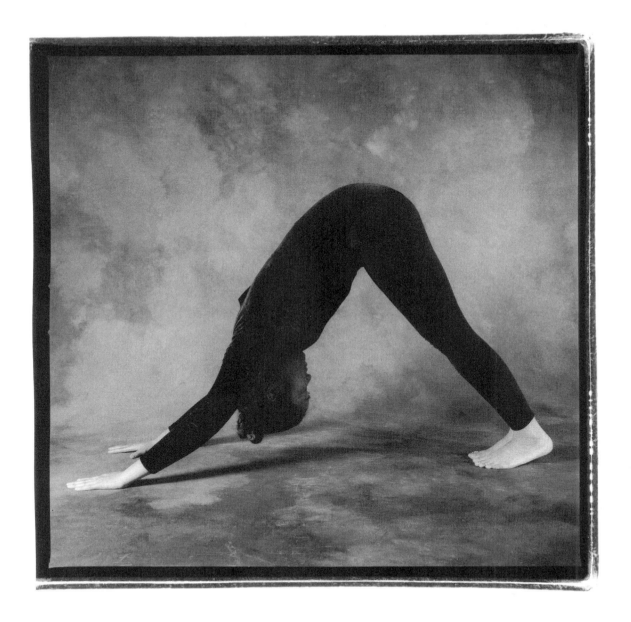

EGG

Over easy.

Follow the Salute to the Setting Sun with the Egg Over Easy.

1. Lie down on your back on a mat. Circle your knees with your arms, and hug them to your chest as you exhale.

2. Roll in several different directions to massage your back muscles against the floor.

3. Roll back to center. Relax your arms straight out to the sides. Keeping your shoulders flat, roll your head to one side as you roll your hips and knees to the other.

4. Exhale and try to touch your elbow with your knees. If you don't feel loose enough, then allow your shoulder to lift as you bring your knees to the floor.

5. Inhale and come back to center. You can add the Minnow (page 130) here if your neck needs more relaxing. Try the head and knee rolls to the other side.

6. Come to center. Lower your head and feet. Straighten your legs. Rest in the Corpse pose (page 86) awhile.

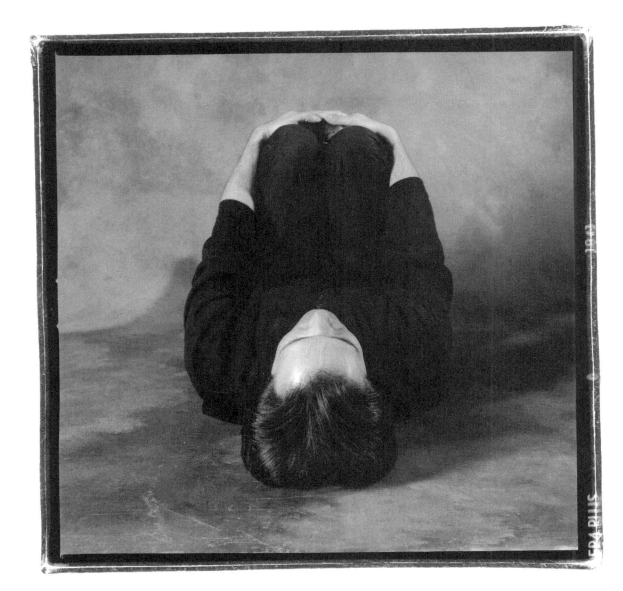

SCARAB

████

A jewel.

1. Kneel and sit on your heels. Inhale as you raise both arms above your head and stretch.

2. Exhale as you bend forward at the waist and lean your torso over onto your thighs. Relax your forehead on the mat and allow your arms to extend loosely in front of you.

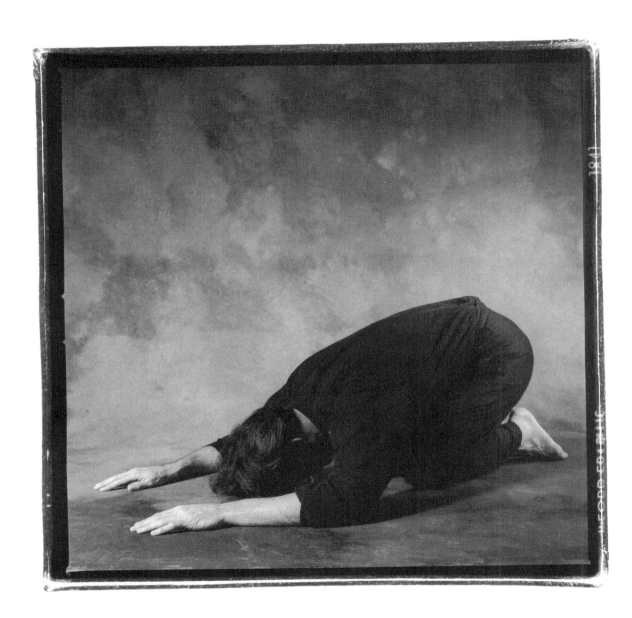

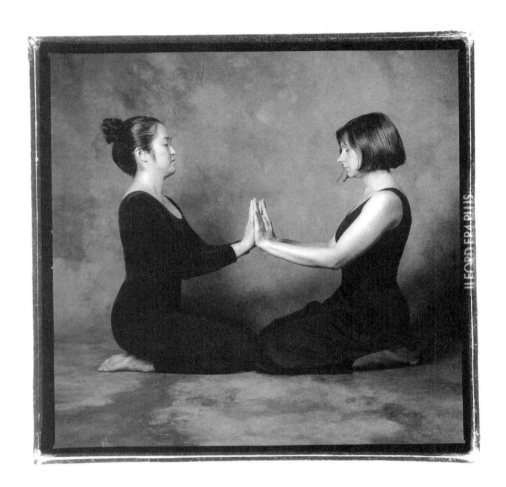

AWARENESS SQUARED
DOUBLE HATHA
KUNDALINI PARTNERS
TANTRA

III

YOGA FOR TWO

AWARENESS SQUARED

The sun and moon are not mirrored in cloudy waters, thus the Almighty cannot be mirrored in a heart that is obsessed with the idea of "me and mine."
—*Sri Ramakrishna*

Teaming up with someone to do exercises can give you a jump start when your reserves are run down. It's fun. And creative. Invent ways the asanas can work well for two.

Partner yoga challenges all three aspects of ourselves: mind, body and spirit. Partner postures are nonverbal blueprints of your interaction with each other. You can discover and work through relationship blocks as well as heighten your enjoyment of mutual powers and pleasures.

Partner yoga provides a transition from your solitary practice to the application of your meditative insights to the world at large. Patterns unfolding in the interactions of each exercise offer a microcosm of your patterns of thought and behavior in wider arenas.

Can you gain strength from your teamwork to move past pain and obstacles? Can you enjoy a sense of self while also sensing and aiding another? Are you willing to learn from one another? Can you help each other stretch your limits? Do you drain or revive each other? When you find a closed door, can you team up to open it? When you approach high levels of pleasure or intense energy from the exercises, do you try to tone it down, maintain, or heighten it?

Yoga is a doorway to more self-awareness and partner yoga can double your insight.

DOUBLE HATHA

Who sees the divine amid the mortal, that man sees truly.
—Bhagavad Gita

    Whether your partner is a lover, a friend, or a casual acquaintance, the exercises will reveal a lot about the ways you function with other people. Some of the postures are simple. They show patterns in how you relax and play together. The difficult postures indicate how you deal with challenges. Either can bring you double trouble or double divinity.

DOUBLE BACK REST

■■■■■■

Reciprocal repose.

Resting alone is healing and pleasurable. Resting with a partner can give you a jump start because relaxation can be catching.

1. Sit on your knees back to back with toes touching. One person assumes the Child pose.

2. The other person leans back to assume a modified Fish pose, arching over her partner's back.

3. Find positions without talking so you can relax and rest together. Hold the pose for a while and breathe normally.

4. Nonverbally communicate readiness to move. Switch poses so that the person who was curled up can now stretch back. Use this pose throughout your double workout whenever you need to take a breather.

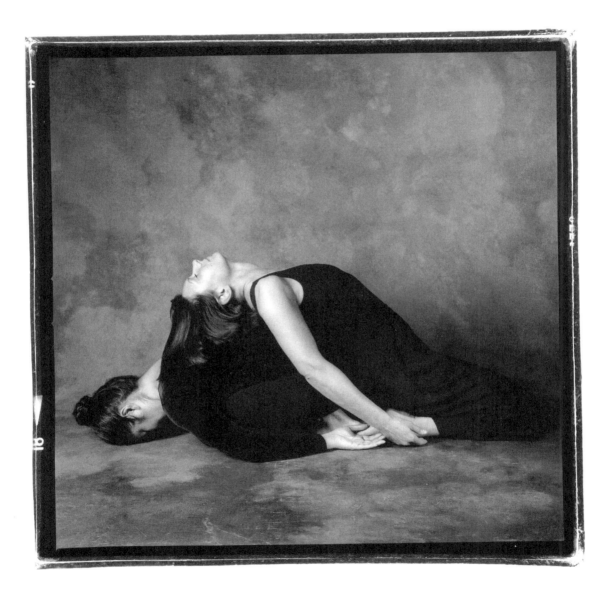

DOUBLE TREE

■

Put down roots.

1. Stand straight, side by side, shoulder to shoulder. Shift your weight onto your inside leg. Focus on a central visual balance point at eye level in front of you.

2. Bend your outside leg and place the foot high up on your straight thigh.

3. Use your inside hand to clasp the foot of your partner for mutual support. Reach your outside arm around behind you and hold hands, if comfortable.

4. Breathe normally through your nose. Relax any muscles that tensed while you adjusted your position. Maintain your balance as you close your eyes and relax more into the pose. When you want to release the pose, indicate this nonverbally to your partner and unwind slowly. Switch sides and try the pose with your other leg.

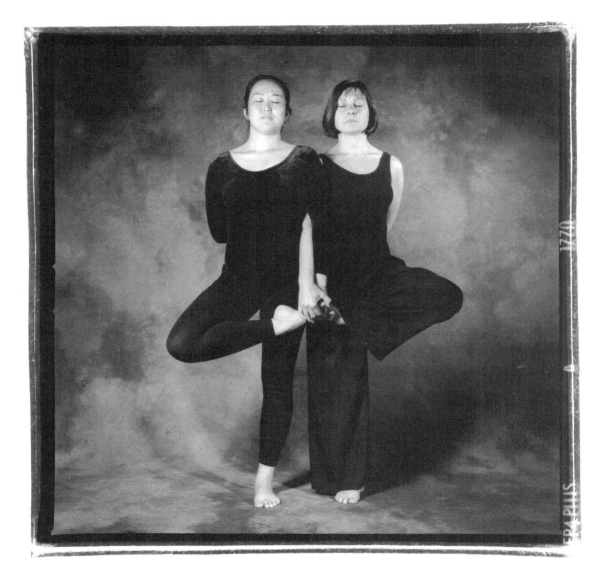

DOUBLE SIDE STRETCH

████

Exceed your normal grasp.

1. Sit on the floor with one leg bent and the foot tucked near your groin, while the other leg is stretched out to your side. Your partner, sitting a leg's length to your side and facing the opposite way, does the same. The soles of your feet should meet. Inhale as you reach both arms over your head.

2. Then exhale as you tilt your torsos to the side toward each other and stretch over your extended legs. Clasp hands of your upper arms. Allow your lower arms to rest loosely on the floor in front of you. Stretch your side and tilt your head so that you are facing front but leaning to the side, not forward.

3. Breathe normally and relax in this position for a minute or two. Release slowly. Switch positions and repeat the posture in reverse to stretch your opposite legs and arms.

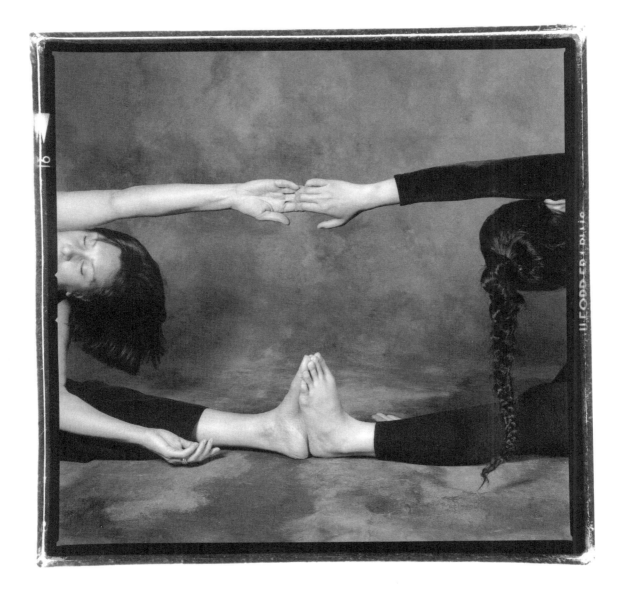

SPINE WALK

███

Sole support.

1. This position is both a rest and a massage for tired muscles. Sit behind your partner, who is in Easy Pose (page 13). Bend your knees and lean your weight back on your arms and elbows. Place the soles of your feet against your partner's back with one foot to either side of the spine.

2. Starting at the tailbone, walk your way very firmly up the whole back, providing support. Linger in areas that are more muscled and press with the balls of the feet and the heels.

3. Return to midback, below the shoulder blades. Place the soles of your feet flat against the back and steady your legs. People's physiques vary. Try to pick a spot where you will provide back pressure without causing your partner to arch her back uncomfortably and where your partner can sit straight with no effort. Be sure you are positioned so you also can relax your back. Support each other.

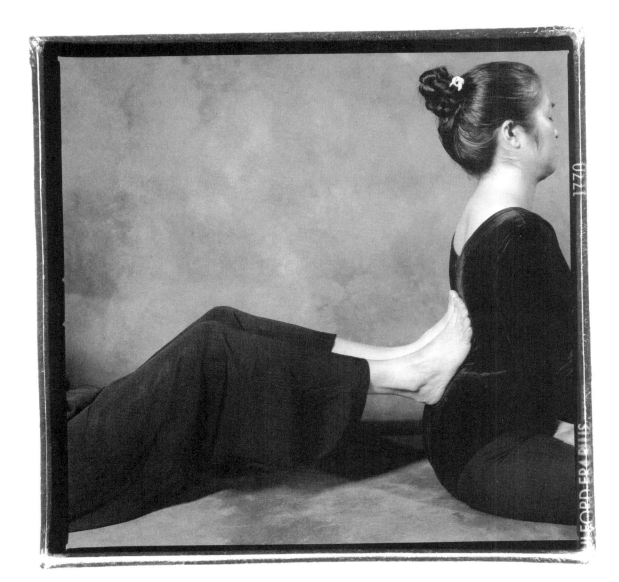

KUNDALINI PARTNERS

There are infinite ways to discover your true being,
but love holds the brightest torch.
—Deepak Chopra, M.D., ***Ageless Body, Timeless Mind***

SERPENT POWER

The spine contains fluid and currents that have biological functions, and in yoga spiritual functions as well. This spinal current is called "kundalini" and its movement up the spine is compared to the wavy trail of a serpent. Most yoga postures involve movement of the spine, because the area contains one of the body's most powerful energy sources.

The current begins at the base of the spine and runs up through the top of the spinal cord into the brain. It is thought that when this current reaches the brain, it stimulates mental clarity. The more you can charge this current through exercises, the more profound will be your mental awakening. At the very top of the head is the highest body energy center, or chakra. When it is stimulated, deep spiritual understanding opens in the person. The deepest yoga understanding is a realization of our unity with everyone and everything.

The human body has one set of nerves along the spinal column to carry messages to the brain and another set to carry signals back out to the rest of the body. The more relaxed we are, the better our spine and brain function, so many yoga positions are designed to relax the nerves and muscles of the back. This helps the whole body function more alertly.

In its complete form, kundalini is an advanced practice with specialized aims. However, simple versions of the Breath of Fire can be done with single or couple exercises to broaden our understanding of the scope of yoga and to intensify the energizing effects of the postures. For further reading, see *Kundalini for the New Age* by Gene Kieffer (Bantam).

BREATH OF FIRE

████

Air power.

Advanced breathing and meditation exercises are fully effective only after you have mastered the basics of yoga. You can do all the couple postures as a beginning student and benefit from the increase in awareness and the physical stretching. Then you can try adding Breath of Fire to experience a new dimension of the work and see the scope of yoga exploration. Eventually you might want to combine poses, mantras, mundras and special breathing after you are familiar with each on its own.

The name Bhastrika means "bellows" and describes the action of your lungs and diaphragm during fire breathing. It involves a quick, forceful exhalation that pulls in your midriff, followed by deep inhalation that presses out the abdomen. You pump your lungs faster than during most other yoga breathing, use muscles more forcefully and apply prana locks at different points. All these techniques increase the effects of the breathing on your circulatory system and your mental functions.

Breath of Fire can be used simply to improve circulation and revive waning energy. Or it can be used in special sequences to raise the body's kundalini energy up the spine to stimulate higher spiritual centers in your head. Used in couple exercises, Breath of Fire can intensify your mutual experience.

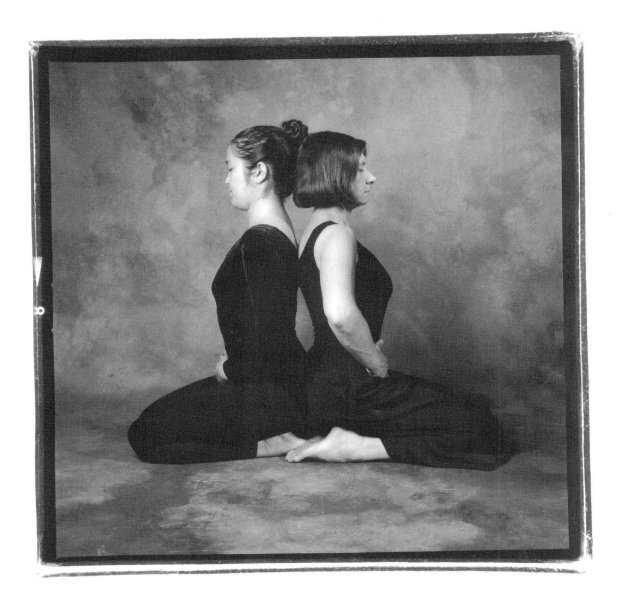

ELBOW LOCK

█████

Find the key.

This position is a good one for a mutual Breath of Fire meditation, because your arms support you during the energetic breathing.

1. Sit comfortably back to back with a partner, both of you either kneeling or in Easy Pose. Reach behind you and lock arms at the elbows. Add Breath of Fire for awhile.

2. You can close with a balance exercise. Breath normally. Bend your knees and place the soles of your feet on the ground, heels as close to your hips as you can get them. Tighten your elbow lock. Now stand up.

3. Sometimes standing up together is a breeze. Your balance and pressure synchronize easily. Sometimes you can't imagine it's possible and you slip and juggle around. If you're barefoot, you can't do this on a slippery floor. You need foot traction from a rug or from sneakers. But success in ending upright largely depends on both people applying sufficient back pressure to propel you up as you straighten your legs. Rise together.

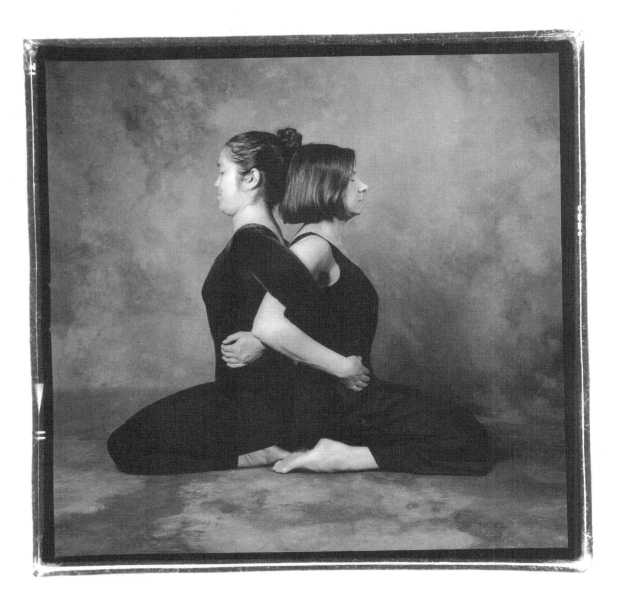

FINGERS AND TOES

■■■■

Touching soles.

1. Sit facing each other with the soles of your feet flatly touching. Inhale and raise both arms straight up above you. Exhale as you bend forward at the waists, lower your heads and join hands in the middle over your feet. Allow your partner's pull to stretch you a bit. Straighten your legs, if this is comfortable.

2. Breathe normally through your nose. Remain in this position a minute or two. Notice where you feel tight and see if you can use your breathing and positions to release some of the tension.

3. You can add the Breath of Fire and hold the position longer, working through the tightness with your mutual positioning and breathing.

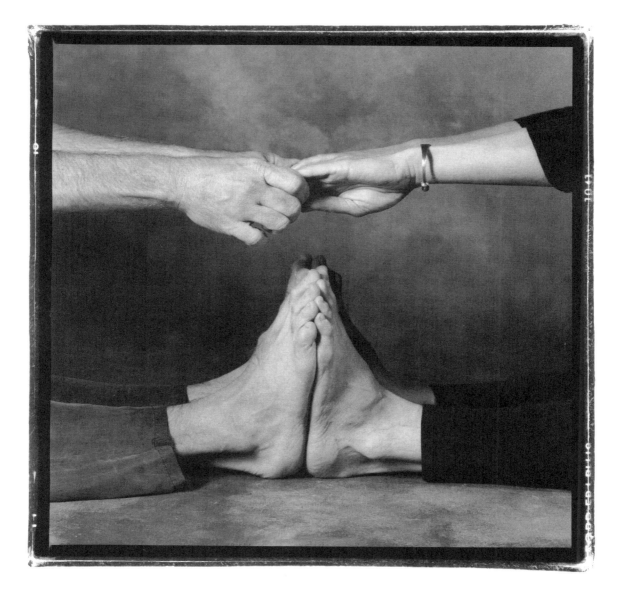

PYRAMID

Power point.

1. Sit facing each other with knees bent, feet flat on the floor. Join hands, straighten your backs and look steadily into one another's eyes.

2. Angle your feet up so the soles become pressed flat together. Gradually straighten your legs and raise your feet, ankles together, above your clasped hands. Maintain your gaze, blinking as little as possible and keep a firm hand grip for balance. Inhale and exhale deeply several times as you secure your pose.

3. Now hold your gaze and begin the Breath of Fire. Continue for several minutes or as long as is comfortable. Before lowering your legs, inhale deeply once and hold your breath to a count of sixteen.

4. Exhale slowly and lower your legs and arms gradually together. Rest on the floor by leaning back to lie down but keep your soles touching.

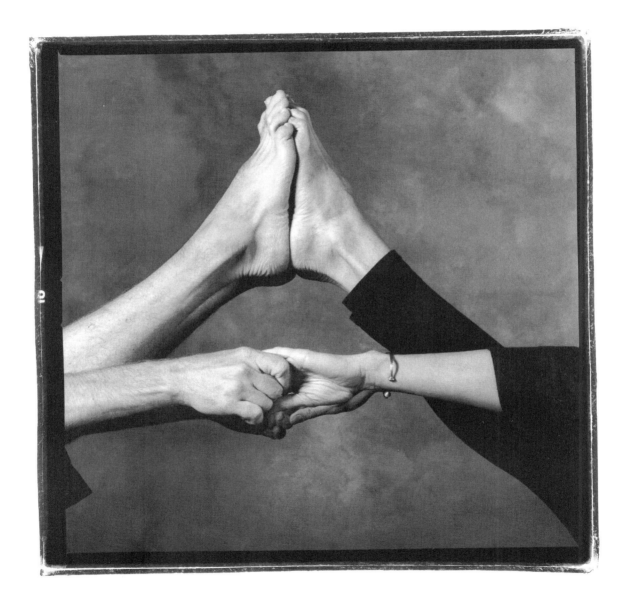

TANTRA

I see all gods within your body.
—Bhagavad Gita

Tantra is a system of yoga that focuses on harnessing the energy in couple relationships to improve rather than drain your physical and spiritual health. Sounds useful, doesn't it? Most Westerners who have heard of tantra assume it is the "yoga of sex," but that is true only in its broad definition.

Tantra is a spiritual practice that includes sexual energy in the realm of spiritual development. Rather than looking on sexuality as destructive to spirituality, tantra exercises focus on increasing your sexual understanding and clearing your couple dynamics of negative patterns. Partner energy becomes directed toward loving, powerful exchanges that raise rather than diminish the power of the partners. Advanced tantra study can involve sexual practices. However, simple partner exercises that anyone can do together can be revealing and useful to shed light on your patterns in relationships of all kinds. *Tantra Art* by Ajit Mookerjee (Kumar Gallery) presents a fine exploration of tantra theory and art.

Mahan or white tantric yoga is based on meditations in which you gaze into another person's eyes. Insights from these experiences can gradually transform relationships between surface personalities into relationships between deeper souls.

Most Western psychology is concerned with the functioning of the more surface personality. All yoga practices are designed to move you to higher levels of spiritual being. Tantra yoga can complement psychology by giving you tools to reach a peaceful state in which to face anxiety-producing personal issues. You can learn to correct personality problems or bad patterns in couple relationships more calmly and clearly. Sometimes you will even sail beyond individual issues to moments of larger spiritual union. These will nourish you all through your relationships.

Two simple, powerful tantra meditation positions are: 1. Lie flat on your backs with only the tops (Crown Chakras) of your two heads touching; 2. Lie facing each other on your opposite sides so your foreheads (Third Eye Chakras) touch. In both poses, your bodies are not side by side, but end to end in a long line. Close your eyes and focus your awareness on the nonverbal exchange.

Any session can benefit from beginning with this Heart Chakra Meditation. Sit cross-legged, facing each other, knees touching. Place your right palm gently on your partner's chest over the heart area. Place your left hand over your partner's right and draw it to your chest over your heart. Imagine that you can inhale universal energy and love from the air around you and exhale it through your arms and into your partner's heart. Your partner is exchanging the same with you.

BACK-TO-BACK MEDITATION

Double your oneness.

1. Sit cross-legged, back to back with your partner. Let as much of your spines touch as possible. Find a position to rest together in which both of you are comfortable and neither feels too leaned on or leaning. Ideally you will feel that the other person's back gives you support to sit up effortlessly.

2. Rest your hands palms up in your lap. Or you can extend both arms behind you to rest your palms on your partner's thighs. Close your eyes. Notice any movement in the muscles of your body as a result of your breathing.

3. Can you feel any movement in your partner's back as a result of his or her breathing, especially in the lower back? Can you keep aware of your own sensations while you feel another's? Notice if your breathing rhythms stay different or synchronize.

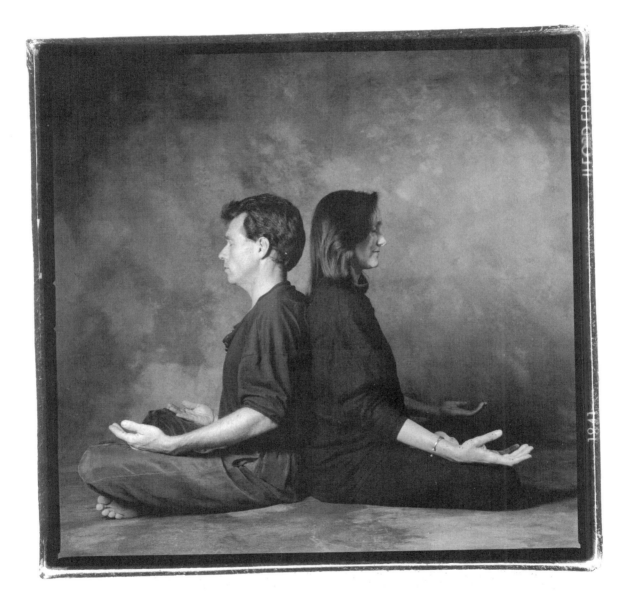

DOUBLE SHOULDER STAND

▬

Heels over heads.

1. Lie down on your backs on the floor with the tops of your heads touching. Roll your legs back as you begin to assume the Shoulder Stand while supporting your back with your palms.

2. Bend your knees and position them flush against your partner's knees above your heads. Try to place them over the line where your two heads meet. Keep your forelegs and toes straight.

3. Adjust yourselves so that you feel some support for the position from your partner. Breathe normally through your nose. Close your eyes and relax.

4. When you want to unwind, do so slowly. Then lie flat a few moments, head to head.

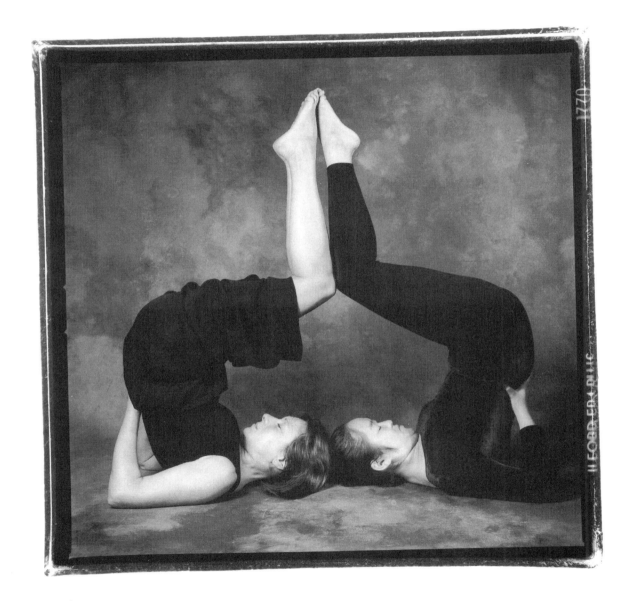

PALM MIRROR

■■■■■■

Electric reflections.

1. Sit crosslegged opposite your partner with your knees touching. Place your arms at your sides and your palms on your partner's palms in the following pattern: You and your partner's right palms should be facing down and the left palms facing up. The four palms fit together in mirror images. Begin by closing your eyes, relaxing your breathing, and noticing how you are feeling.

2. Now open your eyes and look into your partner's eyes. Can you continue to stay in touch with your inner feelings even when sensing someone else? Do not try to talk or visually communicate by facial changes. Keep your expression neutral. Allow your eyes to receive and give information without cen-

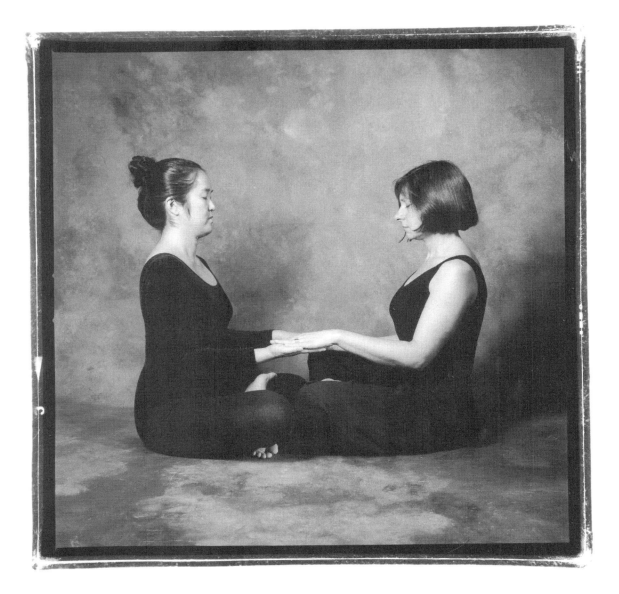

soring it. Notice if you begin to feel any sensation of an energy circuit trailing from your palms, arms, and knees to the rest of your body. Can you relax and allow this energy to flow?

3. Breathe gently through your nose. Imagine what it would feel like if you could exhale down through your body and into your arms and legs. Allow your breathing to ease tight muscles and to relax you from the inside. (A more detailed description of this body breathing is given in the Meditation chapter on Hand Mudras, page 27.)

4. Try imagining that as you exhale you send your breath not only down your arms but also into your palms and even into your partner's palms. What would it feel like if you could send energy to your partner as you exhale and receive energy from your partner as you inhale? Can you both give power to and accept power from your partner?

5. Now alter your position so that the soles of your feet are touching and your legs are stretched straight out between you.

Keep your spine straight and your eyes in contact. Stretch your arms out about shoulder height in front of you with palms down. Your partner should also stretch out both arms, but with the palms up and hands slightly below your hands. Your four hands do not touch. Do you feel any sensation of energy exchange even though your hands are not touching now?

6. Maintaining eye contact, increase the depth and speed of your exhalation so that your abdomen contracts sharply as you exhale and the air is expelled in short, powerful bursts. This clears more stale air from the lungs and allows fresh air to come in more easily as you inhale. The faster pace speeds up your circulation. Both of you continue this fast breath to relax any aches you might feel in your muscles. Gradually slow down your breathing, relax your arms, and lie down on the floor. Allow your feet to stay touching. Rest a while.

TWO CAMELS

A caravan.

1. Kneel back to back with your partner, toes touching. Decide whose head is going to move to the right or left. Both of you arch your backs and lean toward each other as you reach for your heels behind you.

2. Breathe normally. Try to rest your head back on your partner's shoulder. Maintain the position a minute or two and allow more and more muscle tension to release.

3. When you want, lift your head and arms forward. Sit down on your knees, back to back, a moment. To counteract any back tension, both people can fold their torsos forward with feet touching to assume the Child Pose.

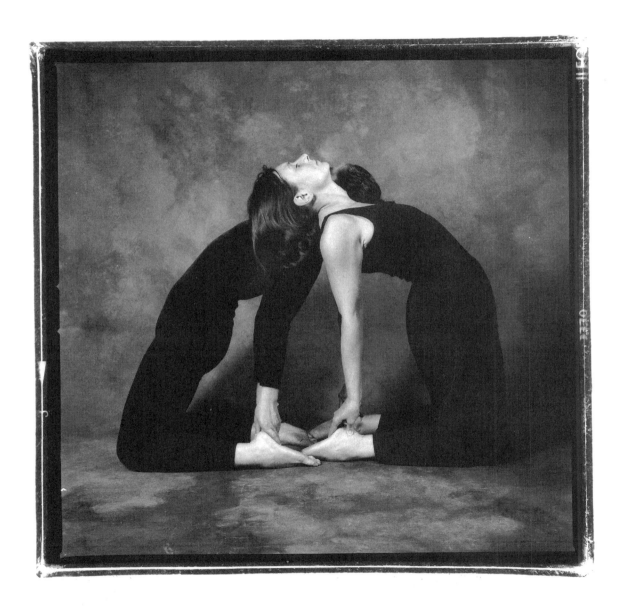

DOUBLE MEDITATION WITH HEAD REST

■

Lean two.

If you've completed all these couple postures, you probably need a double rest.

1. Sit leaning back on each other so your heads touch or can rest on each other's shoulders.

2. Place your palms facing up in front of you on your knees, or facing down behind you on your partner's thighs. Relax your breathing low in your abdomen. Feel the movement in your partner's back as a result of his or her breathing. Feel the response in your body to the series of double asanas.

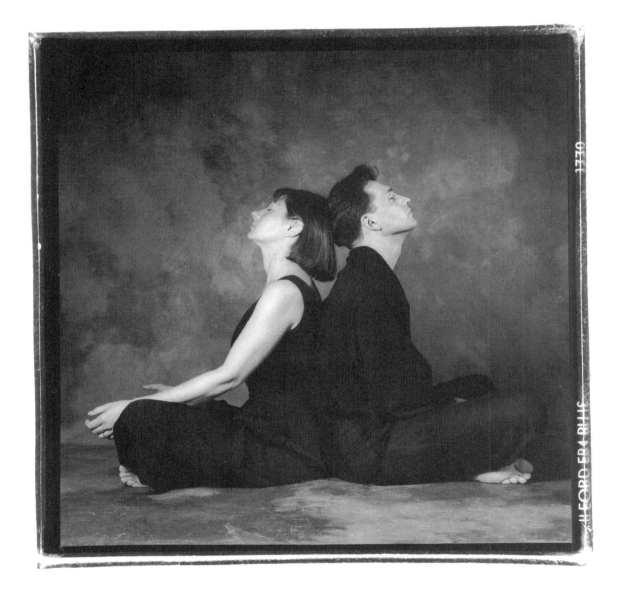

Neither the lotus seat nor fixing the gaze on the tip of the nose is Yoga.
It is the identity of divine unity which is Yoga.
—Kularnava Tantra, ***Tantra Art***

ACKNOWLEDGMENTS

Special thanks to the delightful and limber models:

Susan Orzel
Eugene Ruffolo
Anne Kent Rush
Charles Andrew Scott
Dana Spot
Maki Yamamoto
and Chip

Much gratitude to Freude Bartlett, Susie Glickman,
and Susan B. Jordan for editorial assistance, and to Beryl Abrams
and Susan Sgarlat for peaceful refuge during production.

YOGA FOR STRENGTH, a video by Rodney Yee, is available
from Living Arts at 1-800-722-7347.

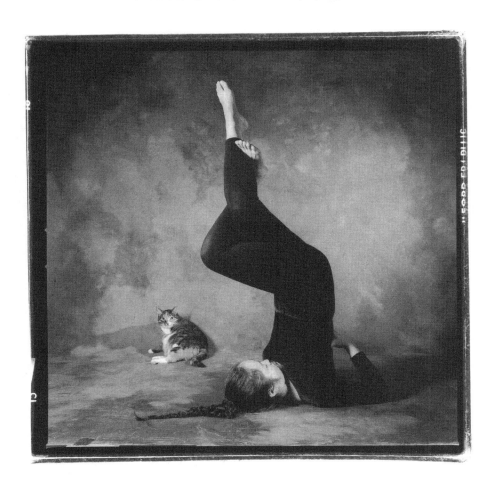

Lose discrimination, and you miss life's only purpose.
—Bhagavad Gita

INDEX

THE EXERCISES

MIND, BODY AND SPIRIT
    Exercising Mind, Body and
    Spirit: Strength in Unity

    MEDITATION: REALITY TESTING
    Easy Pose, *Sukhasana*   14
    Meditation Pillow, *Dhyana Salamba*   16
    Full Lotus, *Padmasan*   18
    Half Lotus, *Ardha Padmasana*   20
    Relaxed Blossom, *Supta Padmasana*   22
    Double Lotus, *Ubhaya Padmasana*   22
    Counting Breaths, *Pranayama Dhyana*   24
    Hand Mudras   27
    Palm Sphere, *Sama Parivrtta*   28
    Chin Mudra   32

    CHAKRAS, MANDALAS
    AND MANTRAS
    Chakra Meditation, *Chakra Dhyana*   34
    Centering, *Manipura Dhyana*   40
    Mandala Meditation, *Mandala Dhyana*   43
    Clock Face, *Dharana*   46
    Flame, *Tratak*   48
    Mantras   51

    BREATHING: AIR POWER
    Vishnu Mudra   60
    Alternate Nostril Breath,
        Anuloma Viloma Pranayama   62
    Prana Seal   64
    Prana Locks, *Bandhas*   66
    Breath of Fire, *Bhastrika*   67

THE MOVEMENTS
    BODY PATTERNS

    RESTS
    Child Pose, *Ardha Supta*   78
    Squat Rest, *Supta Bhujapidasana*   80
    Egg, *Supta Janu Sirasana*   82
    Egg Roll, *Supta Navasana*   84
    Corpse Rest, *Savasan*   86

    WARMUPS
    Fourth Chakra Stimulation,
        Anahata Chakra   90
    Salute to the Sun, *Soorya Namaskar*   92

    FORWARD MOTIONS
    Headstand, *Sirshasan*   100
    Shoulder Stand, *Sarvangasan*   104
    Plough, *Halasana*   108
    Sitting Head to Knees,
        Dwipada Sirhasan   110
    Lying Head to Knees, *Janu Sirhasan*   112
    Single Leg Raise, *Eka Pada Urdhva*   114
    Hare, *Padottanasana*   116
    Ostrich, *Padahastasana*   118

    BACKWARD BENDS
    Cobra, *Bhujangasan*   122
    Cow, *Kona Paschima*   124
    Cat, *Urdhva Paschima*   126
    Cat Stretch, *Pada Uttana*   128

Minnow, *Ardha Matsyasan*   130
Fish, *Matsyasan*   132
Camel, *Ustrasana*   134
Bow, *Dhanurasana*   136
Wheel, *Chakrasana*   138

TWISTS AND STRETCHES
Neck Rolls, *Sirsa Parivrtta*   142
Warrior, *Veerasana*   144
Cow's Head, *Gomukhasana*   146
Leg Joints Opener, *Bhadrasana*   148
Spine Twist, *Ardha Matsendrasan*   150
Triangle, *Trikonasana*   154

BALANCING ACTS
Dancer, *Ubhaya Hasta Urdhva*   158
Half Bear, *Ardha Upavishta Konasana*   160
Full Bear, *Upavishta Konasana*   162
Crow, *Kakasana*   164
Tree, *Vrikshasana*   166
Eagle, *Garuda Asana*   168
Lord Nataraja Pose, *Natarajasan*   170
Standing Half Lotus, *Ardha Padmasana*   172

COOLDOWNS
Salute to the Setting Sun,
   Soorya Namaskar   176
Egg, *Supta Janu*   178
Scarab, *Supta Purva*   180

YOGA FOR TWO
AWARENESS SQUARED

DOUBLE HATHA
Double Back Rest, *Supta Pachimasana*   188
Double Tree, *Ubhaya Vrikshasana*   190
Double Side Stretch,
   Ubhaya Parsvatanasana   192
Spine Walk, *Pashchima Salamba*   194

KUNDALINI PARTNERS
Breath of Fire, *Bhastrika*   198
Elbow Lock, *Anga Bandha*   200
Fingers and Toes, *Hasta Padhanasana*   202
Pyramid, *Urdhva Pada*   204

TANTRA
Back-to-Back Meditation,
   Ubhaya Dhyana   208
Double Shoulder Stand,
   Ubhaya Sarvangasan   210
Palm Mirror, *Sama Hasta*   212
Two Camels, *Ubhaya Ustrasana*   216
Double Meditation with Head Rest,
   Supta Sirasana   218

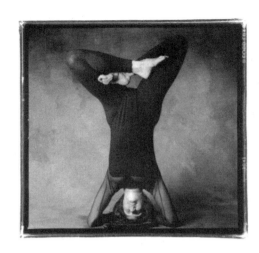

BOOKS BY ANNE KENT RUSH

GETTING CLEAR: BODY WORK FOR WOMEN (Random House)

MOON, MOON (Moon Books/Random House)

THE BASIC BACK BOOK (Summit/Simon & Schuster)

GRETA BEAR GOES TO YELLOWSTONE NATIONAL PARK
(Greta Bear Enterprizes)

THE BACK RUB BOOK (Vintage)

ROMANTIC MASSAGE (Vintage)

THE MODERN BOOK OF MASSAGE (Dell)

FEMINISM AS THERAPY, with Mander (Random House)

THE MASSAGE BOOK, by George Downing (Random House)

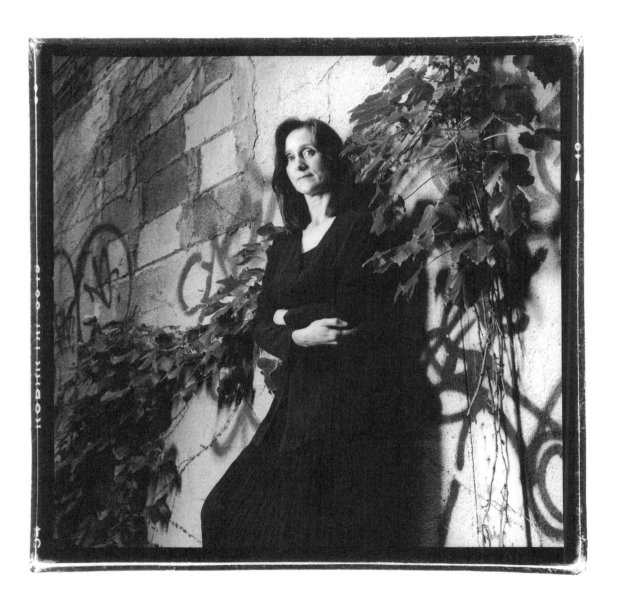

PATRICK HARBRON

For years, Patrick Harbron has been photographing people
for books, films, and magazines. His work has appeared in
Newsweek, Time, Esquire, Rolling Stone, Premiere, The L.A. Times Magazine,
The New York Times Magazine, and elsewhere. In film and TV,
Harbron has taken on assignments for Columbia, Disney, NBC,
and HBO, which have involved working with stars ranging from
Bette Midler to Arnold Schwarzenegger. In the music world he
has numerous album cover credits, and long experience working
with a variety of recording artists such as Bruce Springsteen,
Madonna, Hall & Oates, and Van Halen. Professional recognition
for his work has taken the form of awards from *Communication Arts,*
American Photography, and others. A native of Toronto, Harbron
currently lives in New York City with his wife Dana.

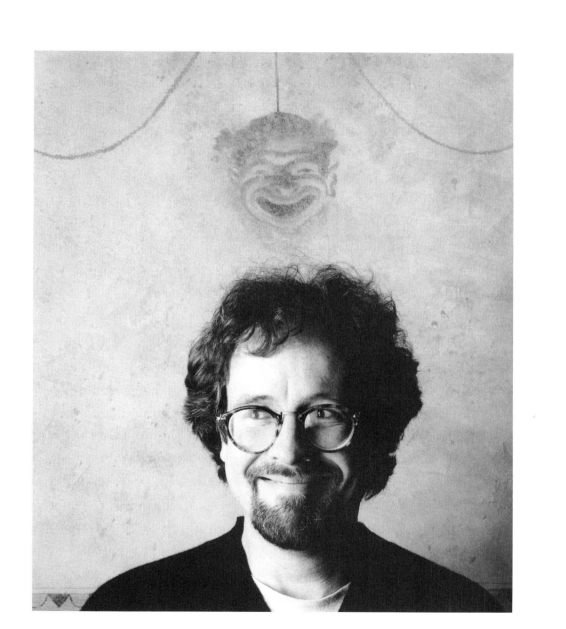

Journalist: *"What do you think of Western civilization?"*

M. K. Gandhi: *"I think it would be a good idea."*